Clinical Behavior Analysis for Children

Adriana Suzart Ungaretti Rossi
Ila Marques Porto Linares
Luiza Chagas Brandão
Editors

Clinical Behavior Analysis for Children

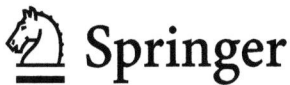

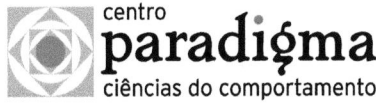

Editors
Adriana Suzart Ungaretti Rossi
Paradigma - Center for Behavioral
Sciences and Technology
São Paulo, Brazil

Ila Marques Porto Linares
Clinics Hospital
Universidade de São Paulo
São Paulo, Brazil

Luiza Chagas Brandão
Universidade de São Paulo
São Paulo, Brazil

0th edition: © Paradigma - Centro de Ciências do Comportamento 2020

ISBN 978-3-031-12249-1   ISBN 978-3-031-12247-7   (eBook)
https://doi.org/10.1007/978-3-031-12247-7

© Centro Paradigma 2020, 2022
Jointly published with Paradigma – Centro de Ciências e Tecnologia do Comportamento, São Paulo.
Original Portuguese edition published by Paradigma – Centro de Ciências e Tecnologia do Comportamento, São Paulo, Brazil, 2020.

This work is subject to copyright. All rights are solely and exclusively licensed by the Publisher, whether the whole or part of the material is concerned, specifically the rights of reprinting, reuse of illustrations, recitation, broadcasting, reproduction on microfilms or in any other physical way, and transmission or information storage and retrieval, electronic adaptation, computer software, or by similar or dissimilar methodology now known or hereafter developed.

The use of general descriptive names, registered names, trademarks, service marks, etc. in this publication does not imply, even in the absence of a specific statement, that such names are exempt from the relevant protective laws and regulations and therefore free for general use.

The publisher, the authors, and the editors are safe to assume that the advice and information in this book are believed to be true and accurate at the date of publication. Neither the publisher nor the authors or the editors give a warranty, expressed or implied, with respect to the material contained herein or for any errors or omissions that may have been made. The publisher remains neutral with regard to jurisdictional claims in published maps and institutional affiliations.

This Springer imprint is published by the registered company Springer Nature Switzerland AG
The registered company address is: Gewerbestrasse 11, 6330 Cham, Switzerland

Preface

Dear readers,

The purpose of this book is to present clinical behavior analysis for children as it has been carried out and to describe elements that we consider fundamental to the understanding and practical application of it. We understand that this is a dynamic field that is constantly evolving, which can lead to different views of the same aspect of therapeutic practice and also to the constant transformation of the elements that make up the therapy. As editors, we chose to preserve the heterogeneity of perspectives among the authors, since such divergences are representative of the current state of the art of the therapy presented here.

We realize that our field has been constantly changing as theory and practice of clinical behavior analysis are transformed. We suggest to all who propose to work in this field to keep constantly updated, to keep up with these transformations, and be able to work better and better.

Cheers,
Adriana, Ila, and Luiza

São Paulo, Brazil

Adriana Suzart Ungaretti Rossi
Ila Marques Porto Linares
Luiza Chagas Brandão

Contents

1. **Introduction to Clinical Behavior Analysis for Children** 1
   Adriana Suzart Ungaretti Rossi, Ila Marques Porto Linares, and Luiza Chagas Brandão

2. **The Clinical Behavior Analyst for Children**.................... 9
   Luiza Chagas Brandão and Márcia Helena da Silva Melo

3. **Child Development from the Perspective of Behavior Analysis** 17
   Tauane Gehm and Adriana Suzart Ungaretti Rossi

4. **Biological Influences on the Development of Child Behavior**....... 33
   Caio Borba Casella and Mauro Victor de Medeiros Filho

5. **Clinical Assessment in Clinical Behavior Analysis for Children and Definition of Therapeutic Goals**.......................... 45
   Ila Marques Porto Linares, Adriana Suzart Ungaretti Rossi, Maíra P. Toscano, and Verena L. Hermann

6. **Evidence-Based Psychotherapy in Childhood and Adolescence**..... 69
   Jan Luiz Leonardi and José Luiz Dias Siqueira

7. **Functional Play: Ways to Conduct and the Development of Skills of the Clinical Behavior Analyst for Children**............ 81
   Ana Beatriz Chamati and Liane Dahás

8. **Acceptance and Commitment Therapy: Interventions with Children**... 93
   Aline Souza Simões, Raul Vaz Manzione, Desirée da Cruz Cassado, and Mônica Geraldi Valentim

9. **Introduction to Functional-Analytic Psychotherapy with Children**... 105
   Cynthia Borges de Moura

10	Levels of Therapeutic Intervention in Psychotherapy with Children...	117
	Cynthia Borges de Moura and Isabel Sá	
11	Contact with Schools: Objectives, Limits, and Care..............	125
	Ligia Lacava Barros and Carolina Toledo Piza	
12	Interdisciplinary Work in the Care of Children	133
	Liane Jorge de Souza Dahás and Tiffany Moukbel Chaim Avancini	
13	Functional Analysis of Interventions with Parents: Parental Orientation or Parent Training?......................	145
	Giovana Del Prette, Caroline Drehmer Pilatti, Laura Malaguti Modernell, and Rodolfo Ribeiro Dib	
14	Family Interventions...	163
	Roberto Alves Banaco and Inaldo J. da Silva Júnior	
15	Therapeutic Discharge as an Outcome of Clinical Behavior Analysis for Children: Criteria and Process	175
	Clarissa Moreira Pereira and Daniel Del Rey	
16	Ethical Issues in Clinical Behavior Analysis for Children	187
	Lygia T. Durigon and Enzo B. Bissoli	
Index...		199

Chapter 1
Introduction to Clinical Behavior Analysis for Children

Adriana Suzart Ungaretti Rossi, Ila Marques Porto Linares, and Luiza Chagas Brandão

In the literature of behavior analysis, a considerable number of publications offer clinical strategies to more effectively conduct the intervention with certain diagnoses (e.g., de Mattos Silvares, 2000; Silveira & Vermes, 2014), but there is still a lack of consultation materials that address practical aspects of the performance of the child behavior analytic therapist. The writing of this book was motivated by the need for literature that discussed these practical aspects. Thus, this and the following chapters compile material written by therapists who share their views on theoretical and practical aspects of the care of children and describe the stages and challenges of the child psychotherapy process. It is worth noting that the population whose care was sought to contemplate in this book is up to 12 years, taking, as the upper limit, the definition of childhood of the Statute of the Child and Adolescent (Estatuto da Criança e do Adolescente, 1990, p. 1).

The child behavior analytic therapist, as the name suggests, has his/her practice based on the assumptions of behavior analysis, which, in turn, can be subdivided into three interrelated areas in a continuous process of reciprocal influence, namely, radical behaviorism, experimental analysis of behavior, and applied behavior analysis. Radical behaviorism is the theoretical, historical, and philosophical arm of a science that proposes to study behavior. Experimental behavior analysis, in turn, is the arm in charge of producing and validating empirical data, by manipulating variables in controlled contexts. The experimental analysis of behavior aims to identify behavioral patterns through the inductive method, seeking predictability and control over the object of study. And, finally, the applied behavior analysis is the

---

A. S. U. Rossi (✉) · L. Chagas Brandão
Paradigma – Center for Behavioral Sciences and Technology, São Paulo, Brazil
e-mail: adrianarossi@paradigmaac.org

I. M. P. Linares
Universidade de São Paulo, São Paulo, Brazil
e-mail: ila.linares@hc.fm.usp.br; luiza.brandao@alumni.usp.br

© The Author(s), under exclusive license to Springer Nature Switzerland AG 2022
A. S. U. Rossi et al. (eds.), *Clinical Behavior Analysis for Children*,
https://doi.org/10.1007/978-3-031-12247-7_1

technological arm, related to the creation and administration of tools for social intervention. Maintaining the dialogue with radical behaviorism and experimental behavior analysis, the applied behavior analysis proposes to produce techniques that guide the practice of professionals working in various contexts, including the child psychotherapeutic context (Carvalho Neto, 2002; Skinner, 1974).

For behavior analysis, behavior is the interaction between organism and environment – be it biological, physical, or social – and behavioral problems can only be understood by identifying the context in which they occur (Skinner, 1953/2003)[1]. Since this individual is part of a social group, this group exercises ethical control over each of its members, through its power to reinforce or punish. Within the group, there are "controlling agencies", which manipulate particular sets of variables, operating more successfully than the group in general in controlling the behavior of individuals. Still according to Skinner (1953), these agencies are divided into government, religion, economy, education, and psychotherapy. The latter exerts control over the behavior of individuals, proposing to deal with emotional by-products and operant behavior of the coercive control, exerted by the social group over the individual.

Thus, the behavior analyst therapist understands that many complaints that lead individuals (or family members) to seek psychotherapy are by-products of excessive or inconsistent control of the environment (Skinner, 1953), primarily the family and/or school. Associated with biological predispositions to the emergence of certain behavioral characteristics, behavioral excesses or deficits may result from group control strategies on the individual. Therefore, to manage such forms of control that can bring harm to the individual and the group, the therapist needs to understand and act on such environments.

Relevant Repertoire for the Child Therapist

Working with children differs in many ways from working with adolescents and adults, so the therapist who proposes to work with children needs to study the idiosyncrasies and characteristics of this universe, as well as develop specific repertoires for working with this age group. The different objectives and roles of the child psychotherapist are discussed in greater depth throughout the book, but it is important to emphasize that when working with children, this professional offers models of appropriate behavior not only for the child but also for the parents, exposing alternatives on how to relate more effectively with the child. Besides acting in a remedial manner, i.e., when problem behaviors already exist, the child therapist also has the opportunity to act on mental health problems in a preventive manner, mainly because the child's phase is of intense development. It is worth pointing out that,

---

[1] The first date indicates the year of the original publication of the work, and the second date indicates the edition consulted by the author, which will only be scored in the first citation of the work in the text. In the following citations, only the date of original publication will be registered.

regardless of the reason for the demand for therapy, the professional should always reflect on his interventions in the light of the Code of Ethics of the Psychologist (Código de Ética do Psicólogo, 2000), as well as in the light of the Skinnerian ethical system (Dittrich & Abib, 2004), considering the implications of his actions for the individual and for the groups of which he is part.

In conducting the psychotherapeutic process, regardless of the age of the client, the therapist has, as one of its objectives, to teach behavioral repertoires that allow the client to deal with the consequences of aversive control exercised by the environment, which are disabling or producers of suffering. In the care of children, psychotherapy also aims to intervene directly on environments that exert control over their behavior and that are producing undesirable by-products. Some examples of these by-products are fear, anxiety, anger, and depression, as well as excessively vigorous or excessively restricted behaviors (Skinner, 1953).

The development of therapeutic repertoire often occurs through classes, supervision, and discussions with more experienced therapists. To work with children, the professional must develop technical knowledge, bonding skills, and management of the therapeutic relationship, which differ from those necessary to work with adults and adolescents. The child therapist also needs to develop skills to conduct the work with parents and the school (Gadelha & de Menezes, 2008; Prado & Meyer, 2004), as well as with other environments in which the child is inserted. In addition, the therapist should also consider peculiarities inherent to the moment of development of these people.

Currently, it is understood that the individual is in continuous development throughout life, but there is emphasis on the study of childhood, since it is a time marked by very rapid changes. Events that occur during this period may have a decisive contribution to the biopsychosocial development of the individual (Papalia & Olds, 2000). Thus, it is of great relevance that the therapist who works with this public knows behavioral milestones of the various stages of development in childhood and thus identifies particularities that an individual presents in relation to what would be expected in typical development, as well as different sensitivities that he or she has to the environment. In addition, since such characteristics can impact the possibilities of interaction of the subject with his environment, they should be considered, because they can facilitate or hinder the application of certain interventions, as well as the learning of new responses during the therapeutic process.

Also making up the broad repertoire required of the child psychotherapist are skills that allow access to private events and the management of operant behavior in ways different from what is done with adults. To this end, tools derived from some therapeutic systematizations, such as the third wave therapies – for example, acceptance and commitment therapy (Hayes et al., 2011), functional analytic psychotherapy (Kohlenberg & Tsai, 1991), and dialectical behavioral therapy (Linehan & Dexter-Mazza, 2009) – may be useful to the professional.

In addition to the skills necessary to access private events, skills related to the proposition of playful activities may also be of great relevance for the child therapist. It is not uncommon among beginning therapists to observe a thirst for information on playful strategies, such as suggestions of materials and activities that provide good results in the therapeutic process. However, it is important to be clear that before selecting any technique or strategy, adequate functional analyses of the client's behaviors should be conducted to then select play, games, or activities that can serve as appropriate auxiliary tools. The play strategies adopted should be consistent with the objectives of each stage of therapeutic work. When properly designed, the objectives of the work with play strategies, the use of toys, stories, and artistic material are successfully achieved.

Stages of the Therapeutic Process

A therapeutic process, in general, begins with an interview with parents or guardians, with the clinical evaluation of the child, and with the definition of therapeutic objectives. This initial stage consists of a few sessions and has, as its main objective, the establishment of a functional analysis that allows the understanding of the complaint behaviors and the planning of therapeutic behaviors. Functional analysis is understood as a basic tool for clinical work and, according to Skinner (1974), corresponds to the investigation of external variables of which behavior is a function. The behavior of an individual is taken as the object of therapeutic analysis. When analyzing the behavior of children, whose main external environments are the family and the school, these institutions are considered important variables for functional analysis and, therefore, are also usually involved in the therapeutic process.

Also with regard to investigating and explaining the child's behavioral patterns and functional relationships, it is sometimes necessary to turn to other adults who deal with the children, including grandparents, uncles, babysitters, and other professionals with whom they have contact, such as teachers, physicians, speech therapists, psychopedagogues, etc. Thus, investigations of the individual's development and of his/her current repertoire, associated with adequate data collection, allow the design of robust functional analyses to then define the appropriate therapeutic objectives.

After conducting the initial analyses, which allow the development of an action plan for the therapeutic process, the therapist begins the intervention process itself. At this stage, the clinician starts with a survey of behaviors that need to be more or less frequent – identified based on the functional analyses – and selects behavioral management strategies that will enable these changes. Through playful strategies, the clinician gradually teaches alternative responses and reassesses the client's repertoire, aiming to develop behaviors that will allow the child to be more successful in the challenges posed by the environment.

The work with the family can occur in different ways, namely, through parental guidance, parental training, and family sessions. These works, in general, aim to help the family implement control strategies that are healthier for the child and the group. In parallel, the school can be involved in the therapeutic process as a complementary context for intervention in the performance of those professionals who work there.

The achievement of the management of the child's behavioral excesses and/or deficits, through the development of more effective repertoires, and the implementation of parenting strategies developed in therapy for behavior control are conditions to consider discharge.

Thus, it is evident the need to understand more deeply some components concerning child therapy, such as the particularities inherent to the stage of development in which clients are, the work objectives, the assessment and intervention strategies, the groups involved throughout the development of the work (child, family, and school), and the skills that the therapist of this audience should develop and improve. Because it is a context with so many peculiarities and because there is a considerable scarcity of literature on working with this audience, naturally, a number of myths and frequent questions about the child psychotherapy process gain space. Some of these myths will be discussed below.

Myths or Truths?

1. The child cannot know about the purpose of the work.
Answer: Myth. Sharing (or not) therapy goals with the child requires a case-by-case analysis. However, it is often helpful for the child to understand the reasons for going to therapy. Sharing goals with the child may even allow him or her to engage more actively in developing the repertoire needed to achieve some therapy goals.

2. It is important for the child to believe that they are going to therapy to play.
Answer: Myth. Generally, this type of interpretation by the child can be deconstructed from the beginning of the intervention. Once again, the development of therapy combinations will depend on the functional analysis of each case, but in general, it is important that the child understands that the therapeutic environment, like other environments, also has rules and that, during the session, there are some behaviors that are expected of him/her. If there is an understanding that this is a space only for playing, the theme may be addressed with the child to help him/her understand that, although some moments may be reserved for playing, that space also includes conversations, structured activities, and different forms of interaction.

3. All activities should be developed through play.
Not all activities are usually developed through play, considering that other behaviors need to be worked on and that there are different effective ways to build repertoires with children, such as encouraging the reporting of situations, role-playing, plastic or graphic activities (drawing, painting, modeling, cutting, folding, etc.), building materials, watching videos, reading books, playing with dolls, animals, and characters specially selected for some purpose, etc. The therapist's creativity is the limit to the development of intervention strategies that respect the moment of development of the child and the therapeutic plan.

4. A consistent theoretical training supplements the need for supervision.

Answer: Myth. This statement disregards a number of skills that are not covered in theoretical training. Supervision will allow a more individualized look at important therapeutic skills to be developed for each professional. And beyond the role of therapist training, supervision allows for support in the individualized analysis of each case and the management of the challenges that a therapist may face during sessions.

5. It is always necessary to talk to parents for a few minutes at the beginning of the session.

Answer: Myth. This type of practice can have a number of implications for the therapeutic work, mainly on the bond with the child. Once again, the decision will vary according to the particularities of each case, and, in the same case, the decision may be made differently at each moment of the work. If the request comes from the parents, it is also important to evaluate what the function of this conversation prior to the session is and, based on this, decide what would be the best format of exchange with them. Sometimes parents may request to share some recent episodes with the professional, and if professionals consider that the minutes at the beginning of the session may be prejudicial to the progress of the work with the child, they may also propose to send information by e-mail and/or schedule times only with the parents.

6. Therapy can only happen if the child wants therapy.

Answer: Myth. No, the child in his or her vulnerable condition does not have the power to choose whether or not to be in therapy. In spite of this, it is fundamental that, if the child objects, the bond and the importance of the intervention are the first points to work on.

7. Therapy can become a crutch.

Answer: True. For this reason, the therapist should be aware of the gains of the process as well as the need to maintain therapy. It is important that the therapy also have, as one of its goals, the development of the client's (and/or family's) autonomy in relation to the aspects being worked on. Therefore, it is part of the therapist's work to plan the generalization of therapeutic gains so that, in the relationship with his groups, the client can sustain the repertoire developed and, thus, conquer autonomy and independence from the therapeutic environment.

8. It is only possible to promote change by acting directly on the environment.

Answer: Myth. Not always. Although access to the child's direct environment is an important therapeutic route, there are other ways to produce changes without intervening in the environment. Many times, in the relationship with the therapist, the child is able to develop repertoires that can help him/her operate more effectively over his/her world, producing more advantageous conditions for him/herself and for his/her group. Through direct work with the child, it is possible to teach him/her to produce the environmental changes that may promote generalization and maintenance of the therapy gains, even if there is no direct intervention in the environment.

9. Child behavioral therapy is just a set of techniques to address a behavior that needs to change, and the same symptoms can appear in other ways because this therapy does not access covert responses.
Answer: Myth. Clinical behavior analysis for children looks at the individual broadly, and analyses of complaint behaviors involve the individual's repertoire as a whole. All behavior is understood within a context and maintained by certain functions. Thus, intervention should be sought both on the behavior that requires change and on its maintaining variables. As we know, covert responses are products of experienced environmental contingencies, and such responses can become stimuli that precede other responses (covert or overt) and therefore contribute to the emission of other responses. Thus, to identify and control the maintaining variables of a given behavior, it is important that the therapist access covert responses.

10. Therapy with children should have a fixed time frame, usually it should only last a year.
Answer: Myth. The duration of therapy should be based on the needs of the child in question. There is no minimum or maximum duration of a therapeutic process. Therapy should last as long as is necessary for each case.

11. If the therapist doesn't have kids, he can't understand what's going on.
Answer: Myth. This type of statement is not compatible with the therapist's training, work, and acting competence. Thus, having children (or not) does not impact on the technical capacity of the professional nor on his/her ability to adequately manage the relationship with the client and the environments in which he/she intervenes.

12. If therapeutic work is not done, the maturation that occurs with development allows different psychological issues to be resolved.
Answer: Myth. Sometimes, throughout an intervention process, parents question whether the gains achieved were a product of the intervention conducted or whether the passage of time, by itself, may have brought a solution in relation to the issues worked on, simply because the child has "matured." Certainly, the passage of time is one of several variables that make up "maturation"; however, if variables that maintain a behavioral excess or deficit remain in effect without any intervention, it is possible that, conversely, the passage of time become a factor that contributes to worsening the problems in question.

The aspects discussed in this chapter offer a small sample of how the area of child care has many particularities in relation to care with the adult audience. Throughout the book, several of these characteristics that make up the psychotherapeutic care of children will be addressed in more depth. Certainly, there are still several topics that need to be further explored and investigated, and, therefore, we hope that the knowledge brought by this book will be a propellant for new discussions, as well as for the production of experimental research, and applied to the care of children.

References

Carvalho Neto, M. B. (2002). Análise do comportamento: behaviorismo radical, análise experimental do comportamento e análise aplicada do comportamento. *Interação em Psicologia, 6*(1), 13–18.

Conselho Federal de Psicologia. (2000). *Código de ética profissional dos psicólogos*. Conselho Federal de Psicologia.

de Mattos Silvares, E. F. (2000). *Estudos de caso em psicologia clínica comportamental infantil – Volume II*. Papirus Editora.

Dittrich, A., & Abib, J. A. D. (2004). O sistema ético skinneriano e consequências para a prática dos analistas do comportamento. *Psicologia: reflexão e crítica, 17*(3), 427–433.

Gadelha, Y. A., & de Menezes, I. N. (2008). Estratégias lúdicas na relação terapêutica com crianças na terapia comportamental. *Universitas: Ciências da saúde, 2*(1), 57–68.

Hayes, S. C., Strosahl, K. D., & Wilson, K. G. (2011). *Acceptance and commitment therapy: The process and practice of mindful change*. Guilford Press.

Kohlenberg, R. J., & Tsai, M. (1991). *Functional analytic psychotherapy: Creating intense and curative therapeutic relationships*. Plenum Press. https://doi.org/10.1007/978-0-387-70855-3

Lei Federal n. 8069, de 13 de julho de 1990. ECA (Estatuto da Criança e do Adolescente).

Linehan, M., & Dexter-Mazza, E. (2009). Terapia comportamental dialética para Transtorno de Personalidade Borderline. *Manual clínico dos transtornos psicológicos: tratamento passo a passo*. Artmed.

Papalia, D., & Olds, S. (2000). *Desenvolvimento Humano*. (D. Bueno, trad.). Artmed (trabalho original publicado em 1998).

Prado, O. Z., & Meyer, S. B. (2004). Relação terapêutica: a perspectiva comportamental, evidências e o inventário de aliança de trabalho (WAI). *Revista brasileira de terapia comportamental e cognitiva, 6*(2), 201–209.

Silveira, C. C., & Vermes, J. S. (2014). Relato de um caso de Transtorno Obsessivo-Compulsivo infantil à luz da Análise do Comportamento. *Revista Brasileira de Terapia Comportamental e Cognitiva, 16*(3).

Skinner, B. F. (1974). *About behaviorism*. Knopf.

Skinner B. F. (2003). *Ciência e comportamento humano*. (J. C. Todorov & R. Azzi, Trad.) Martins Fontes. (Trabalho original publicado em 1953).

Chapter 2
The Clinical Behavior Analyst for Children

Luiza Chagas Brandão and **Márcia Helena da Silva Melo**

Reflection upon the responsabilities and duties of the child-analytic-behavioral psychotherapist brings us back to the very meaning of being a psychologist, forged in the evolution of societies, cultures and which was organized in undergraduate and graduate curricula. To some extent, the way in which this organization occurs distances this knowledge from people and from institutions, which leads them to have different impressions of our work. Within this reasoning, when asking about the purpose of the work of the psychologist, of the psychotherapist, a plausible answer might be "to solve problems." When adding to the question the terms child-analytic-behavioral, perhaps the answer does not change much: "solve behavior problems of children." Such an answer, however, seems too simple, too simplistic, and too mechanical. The idea that the only role of the psychologist is to solve behavioral problems is part of a binary logic, reductionist and hierarchical, that there is presence and absence of problems and that attending the office of a professional once or twice a week can make the problems disappear and, furthermore, that this professional, who holds a certain knowledge, will solve unknown problems that are mine that I know nothing about. None of this makes sense.

We feel called upon, for deeper reflection, to present our position on the purpose of the work of the child therapist. In reality, this is not a question that has one single answer, nor many simple answers. This is the context of this chapter that aims to discuss different characteristics of the work of the behavior analyst who works with children in the office. Since it is a little discussed theme, the content presented here will be based not only on the literature but also on our experiences as psychotherapists and supervisors of services in this approach. It is important to point out that all the proposed divisions of roles attributed to the psychotherapist are merely didactic, since these roles overlap and interchange at all times, varying from case to case and

---

L. Chagas Brandão (✉) · M. H. da Silva Melo
Universidade de São Paulo, São Paulo, Brazil
e-mail: luiza.brandao@alumni.usp.br; mmelo@usp.br

modifying throughout the therapeutic process. To reflect on this, stages of the therapeutic process will be described in line with what is proposed in Vermes (2012). For those who wish to have a deeper understanding of how to structure child care, we recommend reading this material.

Analyzing the therapeutic process chronologically, the beginning may be considered the moment in which one of the persons responsible for the child contacts the therapist or the psychological institution with the aim of seeking help to deal with some situation that is related to the child's behavior and that is negatively affecting the family dynamics. Reflecting on what leads parents to seek psychotherapy for their child allows us to begin to understand the multiplicity of roles that the child psychologist plays. Often, the demand for psychotherapy is raised by the school or by a doctor, who indicates that some behavior(s) of that child may be harming its development and that the support of a psychologist may be beneficial.

Other times, the family itself seeks help because it has difficulty in managing a child's behavior, or because it perceives a difficulty in the child's interaction with peers, or even because it notices a difference in the child's development in relation to other children. Each situation demands different actions from the professional, since families come to the clinic with particular understandings about what they expect from the service they are seeking. The individual histories of each parent with therapy and psychologists in general also make the family's expectations about the work differ. It is necessary at this early stage for the psychologist to clarify what their role is and what parents can expect from the therapeutic process. It is the therapist's role to explain about the functioning of the therapeutic process, which includes practical aspects of establishing a therapeutic contract, such as periodicity and fees[1] and theoretical aspects.

The role of parents in establishing and changing behaviors generates the need for their participation in the therapeutic process, when theoretical aspects will be worked with them. Theoretical contextualization of care for the family helps parents to understand the dynamics of the therapeutic process and can help increase their engagement. We are talking, here, about the need for a posture in the work of commitment and collaboration with parents, which establishes an interaction between equivalent and aligned partners in decisions, sharing goals, responsibilities, and resources. In this direction, psychotherapist and caregivers work in a horizontal, nonhierarchical relationship to design and implement actions for relevant issues, defined in agreement.

Given the multiplicity of possibilities that the family-psychotherapist encounter brings, it is safe to say that one of the roles of the child therapist is to be a good listener and observer. Listening and observation skills are the main skills of the psychologist in general; it is no different here. At the beginning or during the therapeutic process, with the child or with the parents, the professional must always be attentive to what is said and what is not said, since a careful data collection provides rich material for further functional analysis. Based on the assumption that listening

---

[1] For more details on establishing the therapeutic contract, we suggest reading Pergher (2011).

and observation are practical skills (learned behaviors), which are developed throughout life and improved during clinical performance, exposure is fundamental.

In this journey, theoretical knowledge is the compass that will guide the entire therapeutic process, because the professional needs to know where to focus his attention, in search of answers to the questions that will help in the development of the work. There is no useless information, so that paying attention and recording all the information that can be apprehended will allow the formulation of more hypotheses and more functional analyses, whether molar or molecular.

What about working directly with children? To do so, it is necessary to plan the activities that will be proposed throughout the sessions (including planning when the play will be guided by the child), always seeking to evoke those behaviors that one wants to observe (in this first moment of therapy and, later, intervening in a more planned manner, guided by the information collected). Here we find another of the child therapist's roles, which is to know the universe of play and to manage child behavior. Such skills are rarely developed during the psychologist's undergraduate education, and it is up to those interested in working with children to develop these repertoires individually. It is worth saying that, in this process, having the support of a supervisor is highly recommended.

In other words, if you are not comfortable or enjoying the exchange that is happening in session, there is a high possibility that the child is also perceiving the behaviors related to these feelings, and this can greatly harm the development of the therapeutic bond. Becoming familiar with children, with playing, and with talking to them in a way that respects their level of development may be good ways to develop as a child therapist.

Following chronologically the flow of care, the next important role of the child therapist is that of "functional analyst." Doing functional analysis is almost never a simple task, but it is the path to be followed by the psychotherapist who needs to understand more clearly what is happening in the different environments of the child, especially in the family sphere, which consequently will enable him to contribute to the work with the family in a more profoundly effective and more transformative way. This posture is certainly antagonistic to the focus only on the resolution of specific problems. The whole intervention proposed by the clinical behavior analyst is based on functional analyses of the complaint behaviors or relevant behaviors (initially presented by parents and children), as well as broader analyses of the functioning of the client's environment in general. It is part of this process to select which, among the data collected, are interesting for the understanding of the phenomena in question and which are missing, as well as ways to obtain them.

Completing a case formulation may help in this task and may facilitate the next step in the therapeutic process. Although conducting functional analyses is something that is studied since the early years of college, in the initial disciplines of experimental behavior analysis, the beginning clinician may realize that it is quite challenging to perform analyses in the clinical context, when the experimental control of the laboratory practically does not exist. At this time, the importance of careful and extensive data collection is relived, since the clearer the information available, the more material one will have on which to draw in order to create functional hypotheses. With these data in hand, a good start is to create a triple contingency analysis table (antecedent stimulus-response-consequence), placing the behavior-question as the response, and try to fill in the antecedent and consequence fields with all the information obtained via report or direct observation. Supervision can be of great value to broaden and deepen the analysis and to plan the next steps more clearly.

Initial analysis carried out, the therapist should be able to transform a set of functional analysis into intervention planning, to be discussed with the child and their guardians within the principles of partnership and co-responsibility that sustain the psychotherapeutic process. Planning is a task of which little is said, but it is one of the most relevant elements in the development of psychotherapy. Planning intervention is to program in which behaviors to intervene, in what way and in what sequence, and, finally, where one wants to get with the therapy. This planning is, and should be, flexible; since therapy is like "changing the tire of the car with the car running," the child's universe does not stop changing after the analyses are done, and new elements are presented as time goes by.

Hence, one of the reasons why the evaluation process should occur throughout the therapeutic process. Despite the possibility of altering the planning throughout the work, it is important to know where to start and what one wants to achieve. The transformation of analysis into planning demands good, initially, and as the therapist becomes more experienced, excellent theoretical knowledge of behavior analysis – understanding modeling and differential reinforcement, among other concepts – and also how to use them in practice. In conducting the session, the therapist needs to be guided by theory. Once again, supervision can help a lot in this process! It is worth noting that the intervention plan in working with children may include not only the objectives of the work in relation to them but also the parents and the school, as will be explained in later chapters of the book.

What exactly does "transforming a set of functional analyses into intervention planning" mean? The following situation will seek to exemplify: suppose a child is brought to the clinic for yelling at his parents "out of the blue." The parents cannot understand what is happening, but they can no longer stand such verbal violence at home and feel that they are not managing to educate their child as they would like. The therapist talks to the parents, holds some sessions with the child, and gets a lot of information. The analyses he carries out lead him to the hypothesis that the parents tend to deny the child's requests when she asks in a polite and kind way and provide what she requests when she yells. With these analyses, it is hypothesized that the complaint behaviors here are being maintained, because shouting provides access to reinforcers, while talking does not. Only this functional understanding allows us to elaborate an intervention plan focused on replacing the complaint behaviors with others that positively   alter the family dynamics and that do not bring damages, or at least minimize them, to the child, her parents, and eventually other family members.

In this case, the therapist may plan an intervention that includes, for example, guidance for parents and work with the child focused on differentially reinforcing responses to ask in a polite manner, to the detriment of aggressive responses. Such interventions and guidance should always be done taking into account specific family dynamics and also functionally analyzing the parents' behaviors to increase the likelihood that the proposed changes will be effective and long-lasting.

It is worth an addendum on the moment of intervention planning: in addition to functionally analyzing elements responsible for the maintenance of current problem behaviors, taking into account the broader objective of the therapeutic process, of human development, it is worth thinking of repertories that can be taught that are not necessarily linked to the resolution of current problem behaviors but that can be related to the prevention of future problems. Collaborating to care for the context in which the child is growing up, in the family, school, and community dimensions, for example, produces gains for the family and society. To the extent that, as therapists, we participate in the construction of nurturing environments for children and their caregivers, we are collaborating to promote health and prevent health problems.

The field of prevention studies broadly describes risk and protective factors for the development of mental health problems. That is, it describes elements related to the greater or lesser likelihood of a problem, so that it is possible to work to prevent or interrupt the escalation of problems relevant to the individual and society. Thus, it is up to the clinical psychologist who works with children to know risk factors for the development of the most prevalent psychological problems and know how to identify their presence in the child's context. With this, it is possible to arrange contingencies and teach behavioral repertoires that allow minimizing these risk factors, promoting protective factors. Thus, when planning an intervention, it is pertinent not only to evaluate the contingencies that promote current complaint behaviors but also to analyze issues that may arise in the medium term, for example, during adolescence, and plan actions that can prevent or minimize damage.

Once the intervention plan has been designed, taking into account current and future developmental needs, the time comes to talk to parents again and to discuss with them what was observed and analyzed in the first contacts with them and with the child. Here arises another role of the child therapist, the role of communicator. Technical and hermetic   language does not invite parents to dialogue, to collaboration (in that sense that we approached in the opening pages). This language establishes distance and perhaps serves to prescribe rules to parents about what they should do. In this sense, it distances us from the working posture we advocate here.

It is up to the therapist to develop a way of communicating that conveys the technical information involved in his evaluation, but without neglecting to establish the necessary partnership. This – very difficult – skill is necessary from the first contact with the parents, since from the interview the therapist shares with the family information based on theories and research, generally available in dense language difficult for lay people to understand. Sharing analyses and descriptions of functional relationships is a task that can be difficult, since they may touch on sensitive issues for family members. The role of translator of "behaviorese" into Portuguese is perhaps one of the most demanding activities of the office of child therapist. Doing this with empathy and taking into account the feelings of all involved is an eternal challenge.

This moment requires an empathic and sensitive look from the therapist, as well as didactic. It is common for parents to blame themselves for the difficulties their children face. Therefore, the clinician should avoid a blameful tone when describing the establishment of problem behaviors. The use of analogies and metaphors, as well as examples that may have happened during the sessions, can help parents visualize the functional relationships to be presented at this time, increasing their understanding and their possibility of appropriation of the process. These and other resources can be used in the construction of the therapeutic alliance with parents, since, in the work with children, in addition to the bond with the client himself, the establishment of a good bond with the family is fundamental for the progress and maintenance of the therapeutic process, since, in addition to having a significant part of the contingencies that maintain the child's repertoire, they are responsible for the decision to continue therapy. This means that the therapeutic alliance with the family is an important predictor for the success of psychotherapy. Collaborating to build an environment that favors parents' understanding and appropriation of the dynamics of the therapeutic process and the maintenance of behaviors – desirable or not – may increase engagement in the therapeutic process and facilitate the generalization of therapy gains.

With the family and therapist opting to continue the therapeutic process, a stage with a mainly interventional character begins (highlight the term "mainly," since the evaluation of behaviors continues to occur throughout the therapeutic process). During the therapeutic intervention, the role of teaching new behaviors to children through behavioral strategies to help them overcome current difficulties and act as active agents of change in the intra- and extra-consultant environment comes into play. It is important to note here that this role is very different from that proposed in the early days of behavioral therapy, in the behavior modification era. It goes beyond reducing the frequency of inappropriate responses. The application of behavioral strategies here is one part of a much more complex whole. Behavior modification only makes sense and does not produce all the complications criticized back then, as part of constant analysis, which takes into account not only the child but his environment. The behavioral strategies used will be those defined at the time of intervention planning, seeking not only the specific transformation of a given behavior but the change of a broader repertoire in a sustainable manner over time, always taking into account the child's full development and interaction with the environment.

In practice, this role includes, for example, ignoring inappropriate behaviors and reinforcing appropriate ones during play or reinforcing each target behavior in a modeling procedure. So does asking a child to help put away toys and ensuring that he does so, followed by clear expressions of approval. It's teaching the behaviors that you've concluded, after analysis, that the child needs to learn, doing so in a playful and – preferably – reinforcing manner. Paying attention to the child's behaviors can help the therapist identify if the space provided is being welcoming. Good signs are the child's cooperation, smiling, bringing up issues spontaneously, and interacting affectionately with the therapist. In the context of the session, always taking into account the holistic repertoire of the individual, rather than "taking" responses from the repertoire, the therapist's role is to be a facilitator of the child's process. This means programming contingencies to teach new repertoires that allow the child to obtain important reinforcers, in a sustainable manner in the environment to which he or she belongs.

Taking into account the integral development of the child, as the therapist has access to the client's behaviors, he can observe aspects of that repertoire. At this moment, he may identify demands that go beyond the psychologist's scope of work, and one more of his roles comes to the fore: to be responsible for making referrals to other professionals, establishing working partnerships. This is a role of vital importance in the holistic understanding of health and development, since, in many situations, other colleagues will provide the changes that the family needs at that moment. To fulfill this role, it is necessary that the therapist knows the work of other professionals who work with children, such as psychiatrists, speech therapists, occupational therapists, and psycho-pedagogues, among others. It is also desirable that the therapist understands what behaviors suggest the need for assistance by one of these professionals. It makes sense to think of professionals who work in conjunction with the psychologist's work, since this type of partnership brings gains for the child and his family.

More than knowing the goals of the work and understanding the importance of developing these characteristics of the child, it is important to know when to refer and how to make this referral so that the family feels welcomed and cared for. The family may feel overwhelmed with the need for more therapeutic work and may also have the need to control financial costs of yet another treatment and stop seeking help. There may also be, on the part of the family, prejudice and resistance to some treatments, such as psychiatric. Referral is more than just informing that there is a need to work with another professional but a discussion of the therapeutic strategy with the family, listening to their fears and concerns and making sure that the family feels genuinely cared for and welcomed. At times when the referral is really necessary, the child is the greatest beneficiary, and the therapist should channel his efforts to support the family in the search for the requested professional. This situation signals to the therapist the need to work in a multidisciplinary team, making periodic contacts with colleagues to ensure comprehensive care to the child and family.

When a referral to other professionals is chosen, it is also important to inform and explain to the child the need for this additional work – once again making sure to treat the child as an active participant in her therapeutic process. Often, the new work will be with a professional in a specialty with whom the child has no previous experience, so that it is part of the therapist's role to explain the reasons for the referral and who the person is whom the child will meet – always taking care to use a language compatible with the child's development, so that the child understands this as additional care. It is always important to welcome any feelings that the child may express at this time – which may range from fear and opposition to excitement and curiosity – in order to facilitate the first contact with the new professional.

Expanding the understanding beyond the health x illness binarism, seeking a more comprehensive view of human development and mental health, allows looking at the role of the child therapist in a broader way. Health is more than the absence of disease, so that the child therapist can help families beyond the longing for the extirpation of a problem. In line with the premise presented, one of the important roles of this professional is to look at the child's development as a whole, seeking to understand barriers to their full development, and, from there, to draw up a plan with the family aiming at the child's full development. The end of the therapeutic process will ideally occur when therapist, parents, and child understand that the family's repertoire gains are sufficient for the child to interact with his/her environment without the need for psychotherapy support. More details about the assessment of the child's behavioral repertoire and how to work with the topic will be the subject of a later chapter.

Contrary to what a simplistic view might assume, the child therapist has functions beyond superficially resolving the complaint, generally of parents, firstly because resolving complaints by itself demands various professional skills. To do this with care, empathy, and respect for all the people involved in the therapeutic process is quite demanding, not only from the point of view of workload but also from the emotional point of view. It is difficult not to get involved with the situations and difficulties brought by families with whom you work so closely, with contact often more than once a week. It is difficult to find the line that separates the interested and available therapeutic involvement from the "over involvement," in which the therapist exceeds his personal limits to meet the demands of the case. It is important that the therapist has well established his personal values and objectives, so that it is easier to place limits on the work and avoid establishing a work marked by exhaustion, anxiety, *burnout*, and excessive questioning. This time, not only supervision may help but mainly an individual therapeutic process, which may help the professional to (re)know his/her limits and balance.

Finally, it is hoped that this chapter has broadened the reader's view of the different roles of the child behavior analytic therapist, both from the practical point of view, in the different moments of the clinical process, and from the reflective point of view. Keeping a critical eye on this complex role allows us to treat each child and family with the respect and ethics that the profession requires, without neglecting our own health. Being a child therapist demands a lot of work, even more so with the level of involvement and attention proposed in this chapter. Helping families and children to develop in a healthier and more harmonious way is, however, worth all the cost.

References

Pergher, N. K. (2011) Contrato em Terapia Analítico-comportamental. In: Carpigiani, B. (Org). *Teorias e Técnicas de Atendimento em Consultório de Psicologia*. (1st Edn., pp. 135–156). Vetor.

Vermes, J. S. (2012). Clínica analítico-comportamental infantil: a estrutura. In: Borges, N. B., & Cassas, F. A. (Org.). *Clínica analítico-comportamental: aspectos teóricos e práticos*. (1st Edn., pp.1, 214–222). Artmed.

Chapter 3
Child Development from the Perspective of Behavior Analysis

Tauane Gehm and Adriana Suzart Ungaretti Rossi ⓘ

If you are a behavior analyst working with children, you may have wondered how Behavior Analysis deals with the issue of child development. Child development may be considered a secondary issue for some, since much of the observed phenomena could be explained through the concept of learning. On the other hand, some point to the need to look at biological aspects and patterns that are repeated in most children. In any case, childcare settings are generally permeated by age norms, by expectations of skill acquisition related to different phases, and by conceptions based on maturation. Thus, it is important that the behavioral psychotherapist can understand and describe development, or the phenomena grouped under this label, in a way compatible with the radical behaviorist philosophy. This chapter was designed to meet, at least in part, this need. Therefore, in the following lines, we will present the analytic-behavioral concept of development, interpretations consistent with the approach on terms related to this label, and some questions that still exist in the area.

What Is Development for Behavior Analysis?

In the analytic-behavioral view, development can be understood as *progressive changes in the interactions between behavior and environment* (Bijou & Baer, 1961). The focus is not exclusively on organic or environmental variables but also on how the interaction between these variables occurs and changes over time. The

---

T. Gehm (✉)
Private Practice, São Paulo, Brazil
e-mail: tauane.gehm@gmail.com

A. S. U. Rossi
Paradigma – Center for Behavioral Sciences and Technology, São Paulo, Brazil
e-mail: adrianarossi@paradigmaac.org

interactions are always continuous, interdependent, and bidirectional – that is, in a cycle that begins in fertilization and only ends with the death of the individual, the actions of an organism impact the environment, and this impact has a feedback on the organism (Vasconcelos et al., 2010).

The "progressive" aspect indicates that each observed change in behavior occurs not only influenced by current environmental variables but also by interactions that preceded it (Rosales-Ruiz & Baer, 1996). Developmental analysis considers interactions that immediately preceded the change as well as any relevant historical variables (Rosales-Ruiz & Baer, 1996). What is observed, in general, is that previously acquired behavioral competences can become facilitating or hindering conditions for the construction of new competences. Moreover, the functions acquired by stimuli throughout history will influence how the environment will affect the organism and its actions at the moment analyzed, changing the present relations and facilitating or hindering new learning. Considering that historical aspects may even hinder new learning, it is important to highlight that the progressive character has no relation to the notion of progress, improvement, or single direction of development (Vasconcelos et al., 2010).

The study of development is diachronic, i.e., it analyzes the phenomenon over time. It does not, however, remove the need for a synchronic analysis, i.e., a functional assessment of the present conditions and processes that are relevant for an interaction to take place (Gehm, 2013).

The Issue of Age and Developmental Milestones

Although the study of development necessarily involves a temporal cutout – after all, to notice any change in a phenomenon, it is necessary to observe it in at least two moments – the mere passage of time should not be considered as the cause of the observed change (Harzem, 1996; Pelaez et al., 2008; Rosales-Ruiz & Baer, 1996). Often, changes are correlated to certain ages, and, therefore, confusion is often noted that leads people to interpret age as the cause. In the analytic-behavioral view of development, it is understood that changes always occur as a function of interactions, not as a function of the mere passage of time. For example, a child normally begins to walk between 11 and 18 months. This is the average time it takes to experience enough interactions with the environment to enable the acquisition of motor coordination, muscle strength, and balance, among other repertoires and physical conditions that usually make up the act of walking. If, instead of living these interactions, the child remains bedridden and immobile for the first 18 months of life, it will be difficult to learn to walk in this period, even though it has reached the age at which learning normally occurs. From this, we conclude that a child not walk because he/she is 18 months old, but because, over 18 months, interactions were made possible that culminated in learning to walk.

Once this is elucidated, it is worth asking, then, what would be the relevance in doing age or temporal analysis and/or categorization. Gewirtz and Peláez (1996) suggest that temporal units can be used as descriptive, classificatory, or summary variables that indicate sets of responses more likely to be found in groups of people of the same age. In other words, it is a way to systematize which repertoires are expected at specific times in life. An analysis of the early years allows us to elucidate, in parts, how age regularities are constructed.

It is noteworthy that early life is marked by environmental regularities that favor the construction of similar developmental histories among the members of a species. From fertilization to birth, the environmental context (uterus) and the organic conditions of embryos/fetuses are relatively similar in different individuals with the same gestational age. This makes it highly likely that organism-environment/behavior-environment interactions are also similar across all, resulting in traits, repertoires, and learning tendencies common to most individuals at birth (Gehm, 2011, 2013, 2017). Although environmental influences present during intrauterine life (i.e., use of certain substances, maternal health conditions, and stress experienced by the mother during pregnancy, among others) may lead to interindividual differences, including at the epigenetic level, this is possibly the time of life of greatest environmental and organic similarity between members of the species.

During the first months of life after birth, a baby's needs are largely related to maintaining survival. Different infants have common needs, and so they select similar care responses from their environment. Although some environmental variability is allowed, it is still a time in life of great similarity, even across cultures. For example, it is possible to choose to feed the infant on demand or at specific times (variable component), but the vast majority of infants will nevertheless be fed milk through suckling responses (similar component). As in the prenatal period, despite some environmental variability, common aspects promote similar interaction histories and thus similar repertoires among infants, justifying the description of developmental milestones.

The increase in the child's history of interactions with the environment is accompanied by biological changes and by expansion of the repertoire of environmental control, which results in increased possibilities of choice on innumerous aspects. After a few months, the individuals, already less dependent on contingencies especially directed toward maintaining survival and with histories of increasingly individualized interactions, present greater variability of interests, experiences, and behaviors, and, consequently, there is a reduction in age classifications and in the stipulation of developmental milestones specific for each age.

Based on this, cultural contingencies are possibly the main responsible for the regularity of repertoire among individuals of the same age group, especially those provided by the school context. At school, relatively similar contingencies are established for learning specific behaviors at each age (Gewirtz & Peláez, 1996). Such contingencies are usually planned according to a standardized curriculum matrix among educational institutions, correlated to school years (Gehm, 2013). In Brazil, for example, there is the Common National Curriculum Base (BNCC), developed by the Ministry of Education (Base Nacional Comum Curricular, 2017, 2018), which aims to guide the pedagogical proposals of all public and private schools, establishing what knowledge, skills, and abilities are expected throughout basic education.

Therefore, added to a similar genetic makeup among individuals, relatively standardized environments early in life and common cultural contingencies throughout ontogeny produce age similarities. But how important is it to know what is expected at each age? Knowing whether or not a child has reached a certain behavioral expectation at the expected time is useful when it opens up more relevant questions. Faced with frequent delays in different developmental milestones, the behavior analyst may ask: Why has that milestone not been reached? Are there organic conditions that are hindering learning? Is the child's environment adequate to develop that skill? How should the environment be changed so that certain skills can be established? Generally, questions like these lead to useful information, both for formulating a functional analysis and for planning and implementing appropriate interventions.

The description of what is expected in each age group, ideally, should be sought in the child's community (Bijou & Baer, 1961). If the child already attends school, for example, it would be interesting to visit the place and compare the child's repertoire to that of his/her peers of the same class and/or age. If it is not possible to compare the child's repertoire with peers, for the early years of life, we suggest consulting development guidelines or handbooks usually provided by health agencies.

In short, as described by Gehm (2013, p.19), "it can be said that the main role of time in the analytic-behavioral study of development is to characterize the dimension throughout a study is elaborated. Whereas age, as a temporal dimension, can act as a descriptive variable, with which certain changes are correlated, in order to summarize and systematize information. Still, it is critical to understand that age and time are not causal factors." The most important aspect is to understand what occurs during the passage of time. Once discrepancies are found between what is expected for a given age and a child's repertoire, further investigation should be conducted to seek functional relationships and/or physical conditions that may be contributing to that scenario.

Prerequisites and Behavioral Cusps

As mentioned earlier, development is *progressive*, and it is pertinent to analyze how historical and current conditions impact new learning. In this line, developmental psychology has described *prerequisites* for the acquisition of specific skills, that is, skills that, once learned throughout the history of the individual, become conditions for the acquisition of specific repertoires.

The adoption of the concept of "prerequisite," however, is not unanimous among behavior analysts who study development. In Baer and Rosales-Ruíz (1998) and in Rosales-Ruiz and Baer (1996), its use is criticized, and it is suggested that the term could bring the perspective that, for the learning of certain repertoires, there would be a fixed sequence of development. That is, the learning of a prerequisite (behavior 1) would be a necessary, although not sufficient, condition for another specific learning to occur (behavior 2). Thus, there could not exist any situation in which behavior 2 would be learned before behavior 1. But how to prove that a given sequence is the only possible way for the acquisition of a repertoire? In the impossibility of proof, the aforementioned authors suggest that the use of the concept is unproductive.

Gehm, on the other hand, proposes that the term be adopted without associating it with an immutable sequence. According to her, "in practical terms, if we know that the acquisition of one behavior increases the probability of issuing a second, [...] we have useful knowledge. That is, the term prerequisite may be convenient to the behavior analyst if it is adopted *probabilistically*" (2013, p.33). Therefore, any repertoire that, when learned, increases the likelihood of learning another would be a prerequisite. An example can illustrate this point: Kuhl (2011) proposes that sensitivity to social reinforcement and sensitivity to language influence each other reciprocally during development. From a probabilistic definition, we can understand sensitivity to social reinforcement as a prerequisite for language learning, by significantly increasing the probability of its acquisition. Such a conception may help explain not only how typically developing children acquire language but also why children with autism spectrum disorder show deficits in both sensitivity to social stimuli and language. Yet, it is possible that for those children, language learning is established through reinforcers other than social stimuli. Therefore, it would not make sense to point to social learning as a condition that would need to be met for language development but rather as a condition that would increase the likelihood of its development.

Regarding language expression, another example can also be cited. The first words are usually uttered between 12 and 24 months of age, when the child is exposed to adequate stimulation. In turn, *self-control*, an ability related to the suppression of a preponderant response (i.e., the inhibition of a response with high probability of emission – which would be under control of immediate consequences – in favor of a response under the control of delayed consequences) begins to be observed between 3 and 5 years of age (Best & Miller, 2010). Would language be, a prerequisite for the development of self-control? According to Best and Miller (2010), 3-year-old children can already understand verbal rules, and understanding descriptions of contingencies or verbal rules may be important for the sensibility to delayed consequences. Language could then be a prerequisite – a condition that increases the likelihood – for the development of self-control.

Still based on the understanding of development as progressive, some behavior analysts have proposed the concept of *behavioral cusps* (Rosales-Ruiz & Baer, 1996, 1997; Bosch & Fuqua, 2001; Hixon, 2004; Oliveira et al., 2009). The term was first coined by Rosales-Ruiz and Baer, who defined behavioral cusps as an interaction or a complex of interactions "that allows access to new reinforcers, new contingencies, new reinforcement communities, and, as a consequence, new behavioural cusps, which are not always positive or desirable" (1996, p.219). This is therefore a crucial developmental change, which has effects beyond the change itself. For example, when babies begin to crawl, access to varied environments and contingencies increases. Thus, they can reach toys and family members more easily; they can crawl after dogs and develop new interactions with them; they may have their muscles strengthened by exercise, facilitating the acquisition of walking; and they may begin to receive sanctions for accessing more dangerous objects, among other changes. Crawling would therefore be a behavioral cusp.

Such concept enables a type of reasoning that is interesting to applied behavior analysis: "what are the interactions that I, as an implementer, need to plan so that a boom of changes (i.e., access to new contingencies, learning, and reinforcers, among other aspects) occurs in the life of that patient?" For example, what would be the first intervention goal when faced with the case of a 10-year-old child who cannot read/write, has no friends at school, has a poor relationship with the teacher, and displays task-avoidance behavior? The answer to this should arise from a functional analysis. However, it would be plausible to assume that the researcher, based on the concept of behavioral cusp and a compatible functional analysis, would choose reading/writing as the first target of intervention, even if this aspect was not the one that produced most suffering to the child. Learning to read and write would possibly change all of the child's interactions in the classroom, possibly because of the following reasons: (1) make it more likely that the teacher would praise his/her behaviors, (2) make task-avoidance behaviors less likely, (3) allow for greater integration into everyday classroom activities; and thus (4) make it more likely that the child would develop good interactions in group activities and, perhaps, friendships with peers.

It is important to note that the concepts of behavioral cusp and prerequisites are complementary, so that both can serve for developmental analyses. Whereas a prerequisite is understood as a behavior that favors the acquisition of another specific behavior, a behavioral cusp is seen as a set of interactions that largely modify the individual's life. In other words, when behavior analysts question themselves about prerequisites, they are looking at specific learning, whereas when they question themselves about behavioral cusps, they are analyzing interactions that can generate global changes in the subject's relationships. It is worth noting that there is no impediment for the same behavior to be considered, at the same time, a prerequisite for specific learning and a behavioral cusp.

Maturation

Developmental psychology generally addresses not only analyses of the impact of past behavioral interactions on new learning and relationships but also how biological components play a role in determining change. The fact is that there is no development without a biological body, which is in constant transformation. In developmental psychology, the term "maturation" is used broadly to refer to these biological transformations that an organism undergoes during life. Importantly, while maturational aspects influence and integrate changes observed at the behavioral level, behavior-environment interactions to which an organism is exposed throughout life also impact its biological components.

According to this conception, it would be salutary to consider maturational aspects in the behavior analysis' perspective of development. The problem, however, lies in the way maturational explanations are sometimes employed. The term maturation has already been criticized (Gewirtz & Peláez, 1996; Schlinger, 1995; Skinner, 1974) for being frequently associated with *genetically determined developmental plans*, which would define which transformations individuals should undergo during life, despite their lived experiences. Explanations like these generally ignore the influence of the environment in determining behavior, assuming an invariable sequence of changes, which would not be compatible with the analytic-behavioral view of development.

Another problem with some maturational explanations lies in the lack of biological evidences (Gewirtz & Peláez, 1996). That is, many times, such explanations are not based on research or direct observations of the biological phenomenon but rather on assumptions derived exclusively from the observation of behavioral changes (Gewirtz & Peláez, 1996; Rosales-Ruiz & Baer, 1996). Efforts to seek biological bases for behavioral changes have been observed (Tau & Peterson, 2010), but, not infrequently, it is noted that the attribution to biological factors is made recklessly, without the necessary substantiation, attributing, generically, to biology everything that cannot be explained with existing psychological concepts. For example, there are behaviors and sensitivities that are often understood, in our area, as exclusively determined by biological components, when, in fact, they also depend on the history of interactions between the behavior and the environment to occur (Gottlieb, 1997; Held & Hein, 1963; Kuo, 1967). The study by Held and Hein (1963) can illustrate this issue by demonstrating how the emergence of reflex behavior is influenced by previous behavioral interactions.

Held and Hein (1963) investigated some determinantes of a paw-placement response in cats, which is considered an unconditioned response similar to the parachute reflex in humans. In this research, cats were reared, from birth, in the dark (visual deprivation) and, from the eighth week of life, were exposed to visual stimulation (stripes) only for a few hours a day. Half of the subjects had their movements enabled during stimulation ("active"), so that the stripes changed as they walked. The others ("passive") were tethered to a box, being passively transported during stimulation – so for them, the visual change was not contingent on walking. After that, the paw-placement responde was tested, and it was found that only the "active" animals presented the expected response. Their visuomotor experience, understood as the change in visual field as a function of walking, was apparently crucial for the development of the response. That is, specific histories of interaction between behavior and environment were necessary for the development of a reflex repertoire, so that the cause cannot be attributed exclusively to biological factors.

Another example refers to how some "unconditioned" sensitivities are established throughout ontogenesis. Research by Gottlieb (1997) found that the sensitivity of ducks to the call of their own species is established through prenatal exposure to vocalizations emitted by the embryo itself within the egg and/or to vocalizations emitted by other members of the species, whose sound penetrates the intra-ovine environment and reaches the embryo. In the absence of such sound stimulations, the "unconditioned" sensitivity to the species call is not established. Similarly, in the human case, the reinforcing value of some stimuli is established while still inside the womb. More specifically, research suggests that frequent exposure to a stimulus during the prenatal or neonatal period may result in increasing its reinforcing value or decreasing its aversive value – a process known as *learning by exposure or familiarity* (Gehm, 2011; James, 2010). This concept allows us to understand, for example, how sensitivity to the human voice, considered an unconditioned reinforcer, is established through the prenatal ontogenetic history of exposure to this stimulus and not only by maturational aspects.

Within the discussion on maturation, there is a tendency to give excessive or unfounded weight to biological factors. Although, it is undeniable that changes in the organism impact behavior, as well as changes in behavior alter the organism. Considering this, behavior analysis perspective highlights the importance of considering maturational aspects in a judicious manner, based on scientifically grounded biological factors and their interaction with behavior.

As suggested by Rosales-Ruiz and Baer, "[w]e do not deny that biology is implicated in development, that is beyond doubt, but for us the important thing is to discover biology, not to invent it" (1996, p. 229). To illustrate the importance of exploring the physiological factors correlated to behavioral traits, let us take as an example the *stress hyporesponsive period* (SHRP) – a typically observed developmental phenomenon that occurs over the first 14 days of life in rats and over the first 12 months in humans. During SHRP, the endocrine axis known as the hypothalamic-pituitary-adrenal (HPA) axis is shown to be relatively inactive, and circulating corticosterone/cortisol levels are low, even though some stressors are present (Callaghan & Richardson, 2013; Gunnar & Donzella, 2002; Levine, 2001; Sapolsky & Meaney, 1986). At the same time, in behavioral terms, lower responsiveness of organisms to aversive stimulation is noted (Callaghan & Richardson, 2013; Gunnar & Donzella, 2002; Levine, 2001; Opendak & Sullivan, 2016; Sapolsky & Meaney, 1986).

Studies with rats indicate that, in this phase, a neutral stimulus paired with an unconditioned aversive stimulus ends up acquiring reinforcing rather than aversive properties (Moriceau et al., 2010). Such functioning allows greater adaptation to the environmental context experienced by the puppy. More specifically, the duration of the SHRP coincides with a period in which the pup is more dependent on maternal care – a period in which biting, stepping, and the imposition of painful stimulation by the mother on the pups are also observed (Moriceau et al., 2010). If aversive pairings were formed in the same way as observed in adults, the mother could acquire aversive properties, being avoided by the pup – which would clearly bring disadvantages for its survival. The end of the SHRP is close to the period when rats and humans begin to move independently, and therefore it is necessary to protect themselves from potentially aversive stimuli present in the environment.

The organic characteristics of SHRP (inactivity of the HPA axis and low corticosterone/cortisol levels) seem to help explain why pups learn to approach rather than avoid stimuli associated with pain (for a more detailed explanation, see

Opendak & Sullivan, 2016). Delving into SHRP is beyond the scope of this chapter, but it is worth mentioning that the biological features described can be considerably altered under atypical environmental conditions, such as in the absence of the mother, in both humans and mice (see Gunnar & Donzella, 2002). Thus, it seems that (1) there is an agreement between biological development and behavioral predispositions of each phase and (2) this biological development depends on the environment in which the individual is inserted, occurring in different ways in typical and atypical environmental conditions.

Through the discussion on SHRP and its effects on behavior, it is clear that there is an important interaction between physiological and environmental conditions, determining how the course of individual development will unfold. It is of great importance that the behavior analyst also seeks to know the physiological changes and sensitivities of the organism to the environment that are specific to each moment of development, to guide his intervention and to better guide parents on how to conduct certain situations. To unveil the harmony between the changes observed at the biological level and those observed at the behavioral level, it would be important to have more initiatives to integrate the data already produced from the different sciences involved.

Sensitive Periods of Development

As illustrated by the SHRP, there are organic and environmental characteristics that are more common in certain periods of ontogenesis. In these cases, it is not the age that determines the emergence of such features, but age descriptions become useful by allowing the systematization of phenomena common to most individuals at specific moments of ontogenesis. Among these phenomena, it is observed that certain periods of ontogeny are more favorable for the acquisition of specific repertoires, so that learning is highly likely in the face of appropriate stimulation. On the other hand, once this period has passed without the repertoire having been acquired, its learning may be hindered. Developmental psychology has called these moments sensitive, critical, or privileged periods.

Oral language can be used as an example to illustrate this issue. There is an accumulation of evidence to suggest that exposure to appropriate stimulation during early childhood differentially favors oral language learning (Kuhl, 2011). Evidence from cases of extreme environmental deprivation, child neglect, congenital deafness, acquired brain injury, or learning a second language suggests that the lack of such stimulation in this age group, for most individuals, may result in greater difficulty in acquiring oral language. Undoubtedly, for each of these conditions, there are intervening variables that should be considered in the analysis, but in general, compiled data indicate that when acquisition occurs later in life, learning may be deficient in some aspects, especially regarding phonetic and syntactic aspects (Kuhl, 2011; Morgan, 2014). Therefore, it has been suggested that early childhood is a sensitive period for learning this repertoire.

But what makes certain periods of time be more favorable for the acquisition of certain skills? Some authors have suggested that as life interactions occur, organic plasticity and behavioral potentialities become more limited – a phenomenon known as "canalization" (Kuo, 1967; Gottlieb, 1991). Once canalization occurs, contingencies that could return the organism to its initial potentialities are unknown (Gehm, 2017). Therefore, early life would be a time of lower accumulation of interactions, of less channeling, and, therefore, of greater potentiality for different learning. In addition, as already pointed out, some age groups correlate with specific environments (uterine environment for fetuses and intense maternal care environment for newborns, for example). Such environments are unlikely to be repeated in the same way later on. Thus, some stimuli are restricted to certain periods of ontogenesis. Finally, it is important to note that culture has norms based on age groups, in order to deal differently with individuals of different ages – for example, people use simpler commands, articulate more phonemes, and play sonorous games with words with a 1-year-old baby who doesn't speak, which would not happen with a 13-year-old teenager who couldn't speak. In other words, the verbal community is prepared to teach specific skills in certain age groups and not in others.

Based on this, it is considered that sensitive periods are multidetermined by maturational and environmental variables. This is possibly a time in life when there is an optimal match between organic characteristics and environmental stimuli relevant to the acquisition of a given skill. What should be emphasized here is that the behavior analyst should program teaching contingencies that are compatible with the individual's development. One should take into consideration the existence of optimal moments for teaching certain skills, when organic characteristics and natural contingencies can be taken advantage of without further environmental arrangements. On the other hand, once such settings are no longer available, it is up to the behavior analyst to think about how to arrange the environmental contingencies for teaching the specific skill, considering the history of that organism and its biological characteristics at the time of the intervention.

Risk Factors in Early Childhood

The first years of life are usually considered critical for children's development, with studies showing that early childhood experiences may have more significant influences on how the individual develops at molecular, brain, and behavioral levels than those observed in other moments of life (Meaney & Szyf, 2005; Pisani et al., 2018; Szyf et al., 2008). Some conditions, when present early in life, seem to make individuals more vulnerable to the development of emotional, social, cognitive, and motor skills and competencies that deviate from what is desirable or expected in our culture. Such conditions or variables, named here as *risk factors*, may include biological and genetic attributes of the child and/or the family, as well as community factors that influence both the child's environment and his/her respective family (Maia & Williams, 2005).

Exposure to extreme stressful situations (e.g., early separation from caregivers; sexual, physical, and/or psychological abuse; maltreatment; childhood neglect or social deprivation) is considered to be one such risk factor for child development and, in conjunction with other factors, can negatively impact on the acquisition of language, cognitive skills, and on the ability to attach affectively and to regulate oneself emotionally (Carpenter & Stacks, 2009; Kreppner et al., 2007). A historical example that also illustrates how negative early experiences can be risk factors for development is the case of orphans in Romania. From 1966 to 1989, political maneuvers instituted by the then Romanian political head, Nicolae Ceausescu, put strong pressure on birth rates to rise in Romania. Births increased sharply, but families could not afford to raise the children, who were then sent to shelters. Conditions in the shelters were extremely hostile, with poor hygiene, malnutrition, and a severe lack of emotional or verbal interaction. A year after the deposition of the Romanian leader, the case of the Romanian orphans gained international repercussion, and many families from other countries adopted the abandoned children. Several researchers approached the subject, and studies followed the development of these children, who were then adopted and placed in much more favorable living conditions.

Data obtained through longitudinal studies identified that children who were adopted, i.e., placed in favorable environments when they were still young, showed greater gains, in relation to several parameters assessed, than children who remained in institutions. Children adopted before 24 months, for example, tended to have more secure attachments with their caregivers than those adopted after this period (Smyke et al., 2010). Children adopted before 24 to 26 months also showed better stress response, better mental health, and better language development than children adopted later (Black et al., 2017). Still comparing different environmental conditions to which Romanian children were exposed to and their implications, Wade et al. (2018) assessed indicators of psychopathology among Romanian orphans aged 8 to 16 years. Data obtained through assessment conducted when all participants were 16 years old showed that those who remained institutionalized showed higher indicators of psychopathology when compared to those who were adopted at age 8. In addition, the group that was adopted at age 8 showed lower rates of externalizing problems.

But how do risk factors impact on development? To answer this question, it is important to look both at the conditions that resulted in the risk factor and at the cascade of events that occurred between the specific factor and the observed developmental outcome. It is worth asking, for example, what happened between the maltreatment experienced at the age of 2 (risk factor) and the difficulty in becoming affectively attached at the age of 20 (observed outcome). It is unlikely that something that happened in the first 2 years can, in isolation, explain an outcome observed in adulthood. It is necessary to look at a complex and individualized network of interactions to understand this relationship. For example, maltreatment may have continued throughout the individual's history in all relationships experienced by the person, so that he or she may never have had the opportunity to be in a secure caregiving relationship and thus learn to attach more adequately.

The research on risk factors brings correlations between the events "risk factor" and "developmental outcome," not committing to inform directly about causes. In other words, it is not possible to state that the risk factor caused a particular outcome. However, correlational data allows the behavior analyst to be aware of some events that have a greater probability of influencing the establishment of certain conditions and to look at this in intervention planning. For example, when faced with the fact that maltreatment is a risk factor for attachment difficulties in adulthood, some aspects should be considered: (1) when faced with a child who suffers or has suffered abuse, the behavior analyst should ask himself how to organize the environment in such a way as to promote an adequate and secure attachment history from then on, since there is an increased probability that this child will become an individual with attachment difficulty; (2) when faced with an adult with attachment difficulties, it would be interesting to investigate the existence of a history of maltreatment, given that in the general population there is an association between the two; and (3) when faced with a community that presents child maltreatment, one should ask about the impact of preventing maltreatment in the family context on the later development of social bonds and, based on this, evaluate the relevance of preventive strategies.

Knowing risk factors has, therefore, practical relevance, allowing, among other things, a collection of data oriented toward their identification in the individual's history, the elaboration of preventive strategies that prevent risk factors from becoming established in the individual's life and the elaboration of interventional strategies in case prevention is no longer possible. In addition, one can encourage the creation of conditions that favor the development of *protective factors*. Protective factors can be defined as those factors that modify or change the individual's response to some environmental condition that predisposes to an undesired outcome, such as repertoires that improve or change the response of individuals to hostile environments, for example, problem-solving skills (Maia & Williams, 2005). In this sense, studies show that early interventions designed to remove or mitigate the effects of exposure to unfavorable conditions during specific periods of development can prevent negative sequelae (Tarabulsy et al., 2008; Welsh et al., 2007), opening an important space for the behavior analyst.

Final Considerations

In summary, development, understood as progressive changes in the interactions between behavior and environment, should be the object of attention of behavior analysts, especially those interested in the behavior of infants, children, and adolescents. It is noteworthy that, in behavior analysis, most studies with humans have been carried out with individuals in adulthood, with little emphasis on the organic and environmental specificities of other age groups. Such knowledge could be directly transposed to children only if children were considered as mini-adults, rejecting the existence of particularities peculiar to this period. On the other hand, the study of child development may allow the development of more adequate functional analyses that consider the characteristics of individuals at different moments of ontogenesis, as well as more effective prevention and intervention strategies.

If, on the one hand, the study of development can be useful to the behavior analyst, on the other hand, the behavior analysis' perspective can be useful to the developmental sciences. The history of developmental psychology is marked by age categorization and expectations about child behavior, often defining developmental milestones without clarifying how the environment should be arranged for such milestones to be reached. Perhaps one of the greatest contributions of behavior analysis is to denaturalize such standardization, elucidating the interactions that underlie the regularities observed among different individuals with regard to development, as well as assisting the planning of effective contingencies for the development of new skills.

In this sense, as mentioned earlier, changes observed throughout ontogenesis are often attributed exclusively organic causes, ignoring behavior-environment interactions that may, in a complementary way, help explain the phenomenon. In this respect, it is also possible to see contributions of behavior analysis, by fostering explanations that consider the role of the environment in determining change. Such a proposal does not mean to diminish the value of organic variables in the analyses but to include them as long as they are scientifically grounded, also expanding the view to other variables that may influence the phenomenon. The limits, possibilities, and paths of development for different repertoires should, in an ideal world, be defined from scientific evidence coming, preferably, from different fields of knowledge (such as biology, psychology, anthropology, and pedagogy, among others).

Finally, we highlight the importance of building new research that will allow, perhaps in the future, the construction of a compilation on the most important prerequisites for specific repertoires, on the behavioral cusps most relevant for healthy development in given contexts, on sensitive periods of development and their causes, as well as on the integration between maturational, cultural, and behavioral aspects in determining the regularities observed in the development of most individuals of a species. With this knowledge, the behavior analyst can assume a very important role in planning contingencies that ensure favorable conditions for child development, both at the individual level, for example, in the therapeutic context, and at the collective level, in educational institutions or in the construction of public policies.

References

Baer, D. M., & Rosales-Ruíz, J. (1998). In the analysis of behavior, what does "develop" mean? *Revista Mexicana de Análisis de la Conducta, 24*(2), 127–136.
Base Nacional Comum Curricular: Educação Infantil e Ensino Fundamental. (2017). MEC/Secretaria de Educação Básica.
Base Nacional Comum Curricular: Ensino Médio. (2018). MEC/Secretaria de Educação Básica.

Best, J. R., & Miller, P. H. (2010). A developmental perspective on executive function. *Child Development, 81*(6), 1641–1660. https://doi.org/10.1111/j.1467-8624.2010.01499.x

Bijou, S. W., & Baer, D. M. (1961). *Psicología del desarrollo infantil: Teoría empírica y sistemática de la conducta*. Editoral Trillas. Tradução de Francisco Montes.

Black, M. M., Walker, S. P., Fernald, L. C. H., Andersen, C. T., DiGirolamo, A. M., Lu, C., McCoy, D. C., Fink, G., Shawar, Y. R., Shiffman, J., Devercelli, A. E., Wodon, Q. T., Vargas-Barón, E., & Grantham-McGregor, L. (2017). Early childhood development series steering committee. *Lancet, 389*(10064), 77–90. https://doi.org/10.1016/S0140-6736(16)31389-7

Bosch, S., & Fuqua, R. W. (2001). Behavioral cusps: a model for selecting target behaviors. *Journal of Applied Behavior Analysis, 34*(1), 123–125. https://doi.org/10.1901/jaba.2001.34-123

Caderneta de saúde da criança – menino. (2013). *Ministério da Saúde*. 8ª ed. Ministério da Saúde.

Callaghan, B. L., & Richardson, R. (2013). Early experiences and the development of emotional learning systems in rats. *Biology of Mood & Anxiety Disorders, 3*(8). https://doi.org/10.1186/2045-5380-3-8

Carpenter, G. L., & Stacks, A. M. (2009). Developmental effects of exposure to intimate partner violence in early childhood: a review of the literature. *Children and Youth Services Review, 31*, 831–839.

Diretrizes de estimulação precoce: crianças de zero a 3 anos com atraso no desenvolvimento neuropsicomotor. (2016). *Ministério da Saúde. Secretaria de Atenção à Saúde*. Ministério da Saúde, Secretaria de Atenção à Saúde.

Gehm, T. P. (2011). As primeiras aprendizagens com estímulos aversivos: considerações iniciais. *Acta Comportamentalia, 19*, 33–45.

Gehm, T. P. (2013). *Reflexões sobre o estudo do desenvolvimento na perspectiva da análise do comportamento*. Dissertação de Mestrado, Instituto de Psicologia, Universidade de São Paulo. https://doi.org/10.11606/D.47.2013.tde-28062013-161959, de www.teses.usp.br

Gehm, T. P. (2017). *Efeitos da separação materna sobre o desenvolvimento de respostas sociais em ratos*. Tese de Doutorado, Instituto de Psicologia, Universidade de São Paulo. https://doi.org/10.11606/T.47.2018.tde-05022018-150751, de www.teses.usp.br

Gewirtz, J. L., & Peláez, M. (1996). El análisis conductual del desarrollo. In: S. W. Bijou & E. Ribes (cords). El desarrollo del comportamiento (pp. 77–106). Universidad de Guadalajara.

Gottlieb, G. (1991). Experiential canalization of behavioral development: Theory. *Developmental Psychology, 27*(1), 4–13.

Gottlieb, G. (1997). *Synthesizing nature-nurture – Prenatal roots of instinctive behavior*. Lawrence Erlbaum Associates.

Gunnar, M. R., & Donzella, B. (2002). Social regulation of the cortisol levels in early human development. *Psychoneuroendocrinology, 27*(1–2), 199–220.

Harzem, P. (1996). La psicología infantil, el desarrollo y los patrones de la acción humana – Un ensayo sobre conceptos y problemas. In S. W. Bijou & E. Ribes (Eds.), *El desarrollo del comportamiento* (pp. 203–241). Universidad de Guadalajara.

Held, R., & Hein, A. (1963). Movement-produced stimulation in the development of visually guided behavior. *Journal of Comparative and Physiological Psychology, 56*(5), 872–876. https://doi.org/10.1037/h0040546

Hixon, M. D. (2004). Behavioral cusps, basic behavioral repertoires, and cumulative-hierarchical learning. *The Psychological Record, 54*(3). https://opensiuc.lib.siu.edu/tpr/vol54/iss3/5

James, D. K. (2010). Fetal learning: a critical review. *Infant and Child Development, 19*, 45–54.

Kreppner, J. M., Ruttler, M., Beckett, C., Castle, J., Colvert, E., & Groothues, C. (2007). Normality and impairment following profound early institutional deprivation: a longitudinal follow-up into early adolescence. *Developmental Psychology, 43*, 931–946.

Kuhl, P. K. (2011). Brain mechanisms underlying the critical period for language: Linking theory and practice human. *Neuroplasticity and Education Pontifical Academy of Sciences*, Scripta Varia 117.

Kuo, Z. Y. (1967). *The dynamics of behavior development: An epigenetic view*. Random House.

Levine, S. (2001). Primary social relationships influence the development of the hypothalamic–pituitary–adrenal axis in the rat. *Physiology & Behavior, 73*(3), 255–260.

Maia, J. M. D., & Williams, L. C. A. (2005). Fatores de risco e fatores de proteção ao desenvolvimento infantil: uma revisão da área. *Temas em Psicologia, 13*(2), 91–103.

Meaney, M. J., & Szyf, M. (2005). Maternal care as a model for experience-dependent chromatin plasticity? *Trends in Neurosciences, 28*, 456–463.

Morgan, G. (2014). Critical period in language development. In P. Brookes & V. Kempe (Eds.), *Encyclopedia of language development*. Sage Press.

Moriceau, S., Roth, T., & Sullivan, R. M. (2010). Rodent model of infant attachment learning and stress. *Developmental Psychobiology, 52*(7), 651–660. https://doi.org/10.1002/dev.20482

Oliveira, T. P., Sousa, N. M., & Gil, M. S. A. (2009). "Behavioral cusps": uma visão comportamental do desenvolvimento. In: R. C. Wielenska (Org.). *Sobre Comportamento e Cognição, 24 – Desafios, Soluções e Questionamentos* (pp. 387–396). ESETec.

Opendak, M., & Sullivan, R. M. (2016). Unique neurobiology during the sensitive period for attachment produces distinctive infant trauma processing. *European Journal of Psychotraumatology, 7*(31279). https://doi.org/10.3402/ejpt.v7.31276

Pelaez, M., Gewirtz, J. L., & Wong, S. E. (2008). A critique of stage theories of human development. In B. W. White (Ed.), *Comprehensive handbook of social work and social welfare* (pp. 503–518). Wiley.

Pisani, L., Borisova, I., & Dowd, A. J. (2018). Developing and validating the International Development and Early Learning Assessment (IDELA). *International Journal of Educational Research, 91*, 1–15. https://doi.org/10.1016/j.ijer.2018.06.007. Acesso em 20 de abr. de 2020.

Rosales-Ruiz, J. R., & Baer, D. M. (1996). Un punto de vista analítico-conductual del desarrollo. In: Bijou, S. W.; & Ribes, E. (cords). El desarrollo del comportamiento. Universidad de Guadalajara, 203–241.

Rosales-Ruiz, J., & Baer, D. M. (1997). Behavioral cusps: a developmental and pragmatic concept for behaviors analysis. *Journal of Applied Behavior Analysis, 30*(3), 533–544.

Sapolsky, R. M., & Meaney, M. J. (1986). Maturation of the adrenocortical stress response: Neuroendocrine control mechanisms and the stress hyporesponsive period. *Brain Research Reviews, 11*, 65–76. https://doi.org/10.1016/0165-0173(86)90010-x

Schlinger, H. D. (1995). *A behavior analytic view of child development*. Plenum Press.

Skinner, B. F. (1974). *About behaviorism*. Knopf.

Smyke, A. T., Zeanah, C. H., Fox, N. A., Nelson, C. A., & Guthrie, D. (2010). Placement in foster care enhances quality of attachment among young institutionalized children. *Child Development, 81*(1), 212–223. https://doi.org/10.1111/j.1467-8624.2009.01390.x

Szyf, M., McGowan, P., & Meaney, M. J. (2008). The social environment and the epigenome. *Environmental and Molecular Mutagenesis, 49*, 46–60.

Tarabulsy, G. M., Pascuzzo, K., Moss, E., St-Laurent, D., Bernier, A., & Cyr, C. (2008). Attachment-based intervention for maltreating families. *The American Journal of Orthopsychiatry, 78*, 322–332.

Tau, G. Z., & Peterson, B. S. (2010). Normal development of brain circuits. *Neuropsychopharmacology, 35*(1), 147–168. https://doi.org/10.1038/npp.2009.115

Vasconcelos, L. A., Naves, A. R. C. X., & Ávila, R. R. (2010). Abordagem Analítico-Comportamental do Desenvolvimento. In E. Z. Tourinho & S. V. Luna (Eds.), *Análise do Comportamento: Investigações históricas, conceituais e aplicadas* (pp. 125–151). Editora Roca.

Wade, M., Fox, N. A., Zeanah, C. H., & Nelson, C. A. (2018). Effect of Foster Care intervention on trajectories of general and specific psychopathology among children with histories of institutional rearing: A randomized clinical trial. *JAMA Psychiatry, 1, 75*(11), 1137–1145. https://doi.org/10.1001/jamapsychiatry.2018.2556

Welsh, J. A., Viana, A. G., Petrill, S. A., & Mathias, M. D. (2007). Interventions for internationally adopted children and families: A review of the literature. *Child and Adolescent Social Work Journal, 24*, 285–311.

Chapter 4
Biological Influences on the Development of Child Behavior

Caio Borba Casella and Mauro Victor de Medeiros Filho

One of the definitions of human child development related to behavior analysis is the set of progressive changes in the interaction between organism (child) and its environment, in an interdependent and bidirectional process (Bijou, 1993). In this sense, this chapter aims to look at the organism, that is, at the genetics and biology of the individual as inheritance of the species and as individual characteristics for development in interaction with the environment. Along the chapter, it will be described phylogenetic aspects of the human species, the brain biology with emphasis on the prefrontal cortex, the interaction of the organism with the environment through the transactional model, and the temperament as biological base for the constitution of the individual's personality.

Phylogenetic Aspects

Charles Robert Darwin was a British naturalist who lived in the nineteenth century (Ayala, 2009). In 1831, he started a trip around the world aboard the HMS Beagle, which lasted until 1836. During this trip, he came into contact with different animal species in the Galapagos Islands and with fossils of extinct animals in Argentina, among other events that contributed to the elaboration of the theory of natural selection. The book *On the Origin of Species by Means of Natural Selection* was published in 1859 (Ayala, 2009) and had a great impact on the way we see the emergence of the current animal species, including humans. An important point in Darwin's work is that he considered behaviors and instincts biological characteristics, as much as physical characteristics. Thus, they would also be subject to natural selection. To help prove this idea, he studied certain behaviors in current species and

---

C. B. Casella · M. V. de Medeiros Filho (✉)
Private Practice, São Paulo, Brazil

© The Author(s), under exclusive license to Springer Nature Switzerland AG 2022
A. S. U. Rossi et al. (eds.), *Clinical Behavior Analysis for Children*,
https://doi.org/10.1007/978-3-031-12247-7_4

their evolutionary stages, trying to find behavioral traits common to different species. Among the aspects analyzed were hive construction patterns and the enslavement of one species of ant by another species, for example (Burghardt, 2009).

Darwin also argued that humans would not be the only animals to exhibit emotional responses (Hess & Thibault, 2009), which is in line with the current view. Although more complex emotions are associated with the greater complexity of the cerebral cortex, which is phylogenetically more recent, more basic responses seem to be associated with structures such as the brainstem, which are evolutionarily more "ancient" (Damasio & Carvalho, 2013). Decety and Svetlova (2012) propose, for example, that empathic behaviors would be present in mammals, evolved from parental care behaviors. Parental practice, of great importance for mammals, already presupposes, to some degree, attention and response to the needs of the other, such as relief from pain or emotional stress.

Several brain structures are related to emotional behaviors in humans, such as the brainstem and limbic system, including the hypothalamus, parahippocampal cortex, amygdala, and interconnected areas (such as the basal ganglia and anterior insular cortex), as well as projections to the orbitofrontal and anterior cingulate cortex (Decety & Svetlova, 2012). However, the basic affective states and their corresponding neural structures would be analogous in all mammals (Decety & Svetlova, 2012). Even nonmammalian animals have responses that can be interpreted as emotional behaviors (Damasio & Carvalho, 2013).

The Prefrontal Cortex

The neocortex, the evolutionarily most recent cortical part associated with more complex cognitive functions, showed an increase in volume, relative to overall body size, throughout evolution (Fuster, 2002). Among its structures, the prefrontal cortex (CxPF) can be highlighted, which was one of the last areas of the neocortex to develop and, proportionally, showed an even greater growth than other cortical regions (Fuster, 2001). It is estimated that it would correspond to about 3.5% of the cat's cortex, 12.5% in the dog, and 17% in the chimpanzee, until reaching its highest proportion in the human cortex, corresponding to about 30% of it. This increase in CxPF would be strongly related to the evolution of cognitive functions, such as language.

The CxPF is connected to several sensory and motor cortical areas, as well as to subcortical structures, receiving information and being able to influence these areas (Fuster, 2001; Miller, 2000). Thus, it constitutes a necessary framework for the performance of more complex behaviors. This cortex is associated with activities that require greater integration and cognitive control, such as memory, planning, decision-making, inhibitory control, and execution of actions (Carlen, 2017; Fuster, 2001).

According to Emond et al. (2009), it can be subdivided into three smaller areas: ventro-orbital, medial, and dorsolateral. The first two, with connections to the brainstem and limbic system, have a role in the control of instincts, impulses, and emotional behaviors (Fuster, 2001). The dorsolateral CxPF, on the other hand, would be associated with temporal organization functions of behavior, such as temporally integrating the necessary information to achieve a certain goal. For this, it uses the operational memory and the preparatory *set* for action, articulating retention and protension, which is necessary for the various spheres of behavior, such as speech (Fuster, 2001).

As occurred in the development of the species, the CxPF is also one of the last structures to complete its development throughout the life of the individual, according to parameters such as cortical thickness, white and gray matter volume, synaptic density, and degree of development of dendrites (Fuster, 2001; Teffer & Semendeferi, 2012). Brain areas associated with sensory functions develop first, followed by the temporal and parietal cortex, which act in the association of these sensory stimuli. Areas associated with more complex cognitive functions, such as the CxPF, will develop only later (Hsu & Jaeggi, 2014). In this cortex, the volume of gray matter reaches a peak between 4 and 12 years of age, with a decline after that age, while the volume of white matter is only expected to peak in early adulthood, later milestones than those reached by other cortical areas (Fuster, 2002). The increase in white matter volume is mainly due to the myelination of cortical-cortical axons, which seems to be strongly associated with cognitive development in childhood, by increasing the speed of information conduction (Fuster, 2002). Throughout development, the child acquires greater ability to focus attention on a task, inhibit impulses, and improve self-control. This is impaired in some conditions, such as attention deficit hyperactivity disorder (ADHD). In this condition, there is a deficit of inhibitory control, manifested by distractibility, impulsivity, and hyperactivity. Some associate it with a delay in CxPF maturation (Fuster, 2002; Shaw et al., 2007), but in most cases, many changes persist even in adulthood, such as hypoactivation of brain circuits involving CxPF (Faraone et al., 2015). In activities that test inhibitory control, for example, there is hypoactivation of fronto-striatal, frontoparietal, and ventral circuits (Faraone et al., 2015).

Another psychiatric condition that is associated with changes in CxPF is the autistic spectrum disorder (ASD) (Teffer & Semendeferi, 2012). In the first years of life, the brains of individuals with ASD are larger than those of typically developing children. This increased growth occurs mainly in the frontal lobes, including the CxPF, and temporal lobes (Teffer & Semendeferi, 2012). However, the brain growth rate of children with ASD slows down later, so that it ends up reaching a size similar to (or even slightly smaller than) that of individuals without ASD (Teffer & Semendeferi, 2012). In a study by Carper and Courchesne (2005), for example, a 10% growth in the volume of the dorsolateral CxPF was documented in children with ASD between 2 and 9 years old versus 48% in controls. Alterations in neurogenesis and neuronal migration have already been identified in the development of these individuals, which could be associated with these changes in volume increase (Teffer & Semendeferi, 2012). It is assumed that this increased growth would be related to the establishment of abnormal patterns of intracerebral connectivity, which in turn would be related to the characteristic behaviors of this disorder, such as changes in socialization and repetitive behaviors.

The Organism and the Environment

Darwin played a very important role in identifying the theory of natural selection to help understand the emergence of the various animal species that exist today, as well as the evolutionary patterns. Another very important step was taken by the studies in genetics by Mendel, also in the nineteenth century, which were "rediscovered" and gained greater emphasis in the early twentieth century (Boero, 2015). Aristotle believed that the environment was responsible for the formation of the individual phenotype, which would be transmitted to their descendants (Burggren & Crews, 2014). Currently we know how important genetics is in this aspect, including when we are dealing with human behavior (Burghardt, 2009). It is through the interrelationships between genetics and environment that these patterns are established.

Thinking about the importance of these exchanges between organism and environment, Sameroff and Chandler proposed the transactional model of development in 1975 (*apud* Sameroff, 2009), based on concepts of dialectical philosophy and the "nature x nurture" debate, i.e., the debate between what would be innate and biologically determined and the environmental influences (Sameroff, 2009). According to this model, child development would be based on reciprocal and dynamic interactions between the organism (the child) and the environment, placing great emphasis on the bidirectional influence between these two aspects (Sameroff, 2009). The relevance of this model lies in considering both the importance of the individual and the environment for development and in recognizing how one is an agent of change for the other, both being interdependent. Thus, development is not the product of only one (individual) or another (environment) in isolation but the interaction between both. An example that Sameroff and MacKenzie (2003) bring:

> Consider a generally calm mother who has become a little anxious after a complicated labor. Her anxiety in the first few months of the baby's life influences her to be fickle and less appropriate in her interactions with the child. In response to this inconsistency, the baby may develop some irregularities in her eating and sleeping patterns that give the appearance of a difficult temperament. This difficult temperament diminishes parenting pleasure, so the mother spends less time with the child. If she or other caregivers are not actively interacting with the child and especially not talking to the infant, the child may score poorly on later language tests in preschool and be less socially mature. (Sameroff & MacKenzie, 2003, p.17).

This example shows how a difficulty can arise from the interaction between organism and environment, which may not adapt to each other. This interaction between parenting and more innate characteristics of the individual (temperament) will be further explored later in the chapter.

The study of the reciprocal influences between organism and environment also deepened with the studies of epigenetics. This was a term originally proposed in 1942 by embryologist Conrad Waddington to describe the processes that lie between the genotype (gene sequence) and the emergence of the phenotype (appearance of the organism, including not only physical characteristics but also behaviors). Subsequently, its use came to refer more precisely to changes in gene transcription that would not be tributary to alteration in the sequence of DNA bases, with the early twenty-first century seeing a major advance in research in this field (Deichmann, 2016). These changes can be transmitted by mitosis and/or meiosis and are extremely frequent – they are the epigenetic processes, for example, that lead to the differentiation of all cells of the organism from the zygote (Gonzalez-Pardo & Perez Alvarez, 2013). Through knowledge of these epigenetic processes, we can better understand the effect of the environment on our behaviors from genetic modifications. Our gene expression and, consequently, our brain development and behaviors come from our genetic sequence. On the other hand, our behaviors and our experiences end up altering, through epigenetics, the gene expression, thus having an impact on our brain development (Nigg, 2016), according to the transactional model.

Different epigenetic mechanisms have already been described. The most studied currently are DNA methylation, histone modification, and synthesis of small RNA fragments that interfere with DNA transcription (Gonzalez-Pardo & Perez Alvarez, 2013). DNA methylation consists of the binding of a methyl group on certain parts of its molecule (cytosine), which generally causes the corresponding gene to be "silenced" (i.e., not transcribed) (Bani-Fatemi et al., 2015). Histones are proteins around which DNA molecules coil for clustering on chromatin. Histones can undergo different processes (such as methylation, acetylation, and phosphorylation), which alter the structural conformation of DNA, thus influencing gene transcription. In the case of acetylation, for example, an acetyl radical is attached to the histone, which makes the DNA less "condensed" and, therefore, can be transcribed more easily – that is, the corresponding gene is "activated." The opposite occurs with histone methylation (Bani-Fatemi et al., 2015). The third method occurs by producing small molecules of noncoding RNA (which is not transcribed into proteins) that interfere with the production and action of messenger RNA (i.e., the RNA that would be "read" for protein production) (Bani-Fatemi et al., 2015).

These epigenetic influences may occur throughout the life span, but are more marked in the developmental period, especially in the prenatal period. Factors such as maternal stress, diet and substance use by the mother during pregnancy, and age of the parents, among others, can cause epigenetic changes in the cells of the developing embryo, with a potential impact for the rest of its life (Nigg, 2016). Postnatal epigenetic changes can occur in neurons, potentially having a major impact on the individual's behavior. These changes are involved both in physiological processes in the body, such as changes in brain protein production necessary for memory formation and learning, and in mental disorders such as schizophrenia or substance addiction (Gonzalez-Pardo & Perez Alvarez, 2013). There is even the field of "behavioral epigenetics," which focuses on this influence of the environment on behavior through epigenetic changes (Gonzalez-Pardo & Perez Alvarez, 2013).

An important study in this field was that of Weaver et al. (2004), which demonstrated epigenetic changes in the brains of rats according to the behavior of the females that raised them, whether "adoptive" or not – the offspring raised by mothers with fewer "maternal" behaviors, such as licking, had a different degree of DNA methylation of the glucocorticoid receptor gene promoter, which leads to lower production of this receptor. As a result, they become less sensitive to the negative *feedback* by corticosterone, so that their serum levels in stressful situations end up being higher than those of mice raised with mothers with caring behaviors. This was an important demonstration that the psychosocial environment present early in life has an impact on the stress response in adulthood. These methylation effects could also be reversed with intracerebral administration of certain substances, showing that these changes were not definitive.

The Temperament

Temperament is a well-established concept in child and adolescent psychology and psychiatry for decades from studies by Thomas et al. (1963). These researchers described temperament as the child's "style" of behavioral response to different stimuli in different environments (Thomas & Chess, 1977). Rothbart and his team (Rothbart & Ahadi, 1994) extended the concept of temperament, describing it as the unique set of constitutional characteristics that describe the difference in individual **reactivity** and **self-regulation** in the face of external and internal stimuli. These characteristics (a) are innate and biological in that they are present from birth (with both genetic and intrauterine environmental etiology with epigenetic influence), (b) tend to be stable over time in different environmental situations, (c) suffer both biological and environmental influences throughout development, and (d) interact with the environment, having a primary function in the individual's adaptation (Rothbart & Ahadi, 1994).

Temperament, then, is the emotional basis of the individual for continuous and complex interaction with the environment, until the consolidation of personality in adulthood, from temperamental core traits. As the child grows up, it is a challenge to separate temperamental traits from his or her personality built by learning in interaction with the environment, even more so considering that the same temperamental dispositions may express themselves in different ways depending on age. For example, prospective studies have shown that 4-month-old children with intense negative motor and emotional responses of fear and frustration to novel stimuli had, at age 3, a greater chance of introversion and, at school age, greater shyness and social isolation (Fox et al., 2005). Although there is a temporal continuum between emotional responses, it is a challenge to infer the weight of both temperament, as a biological constitution, and the environment in the observed traits to maintain or change behavioral patterns. Next, we detail temperament concepts based on the concepts described by Rothbart and his team (1994).

Reactivity is defined by the pattern of emotional, motor, and attentional responses (or excitability) of the individual to an internal (the body itself) or external stimulus (Rothbart & Ahadi, 1994). These responses have a significant biological component: the changes are physiological both in the brain (central nervous system) and in other organs of the body (such as heart and respiratory rate, gastric sensations and satiety, body temperature, and sweating) regulated by branches of the nervous system, called the peripheral nervous system. Thus, reactivity as a biological and somatic experience (of body sensations) is one of the primary elements for the constitution of emotional and, therefore, behavioral responses.

Reactivity is divided into **activity** (intensity of motor and verbal activity) and **emotionality** (intensity of emotional experience and expression). Emotionality can be divided into "positive" (e.g., joy) and "negative" (e.g., anger or fear) (Rothbart & Ahadi, 1994). Imagine a simple situation: a 12-month-old child facing a novel external stimulus (such as a noisy toy). This child's reactivity would be defined by the pattern, in front of the toy, of (a) attentional response (ability to perceive the new stimulus), (b) emotional response (physiological reactions with expressed characteristics that we name as "joy," "enthusiasm," "fear," or "anger," for example), and (c) motor response (walking, running, moving or standing still, talking, or being quiet).

The quantitative measures used in research to investigate the described components of **reactivity** are reactional threshold and latency, intensity, time to peak reactivity, and time to recovery from the individual's baseline state (Rothbart & Ahadi, 1994). **Reactivity**, therefore, comprises characteristics that help differentiate the quality and quantity of children's behavioral responses. Imagine two 12-month-old children with the same fear reaction, with crying and motor agitation with running away from a scary toy. Even with similar reactions, the two children's reactivity may have markedly different characteristics, with distinct thresholds (the amount of noise made by the toy to activate fear with crying and agitation), latencies (the time until crying begins), intensities (the amount of screaming and motor activity associated with crying), times to peak reaction (time to the most intense crying), and times to recovery (to return to baseline described as "calm").

Self-regulation refers to the modulation of reactivity, that is, the individual's own capacity to interfere and control innate reactions through regulatory brain processes (Rothbart & Ahadi, 1994). These processes include focus and attentional persistence, attentional alternation, and inhibitory control. Thus, in the face of initial emotional reactions, it is possible to observe self-regulation through a child's ability to return to its baseline state and control its **reactivity**. The self-regulatory capacity emerges from the first months of life and continues to develop for years, with a strong influence of environmental learning (Posner & Rothbart, 1998).

Measures of Temperament

Rothbart's temperamental model, initially developed to describe behavioral responses in infants, was expanded and today describes and quantifies, by means of validated questionnaires with dimensional measures, from newborns to adults (Rothbart et al., 2001). Factorial analyses of the different age groups show three dimensions that aggregate different temperamental factors, common to all ages: negative affect (reactivity related to negative emotionality), extroversion/positive affect (surgency, reactivity associated with motor activity, and positive emotionality), and effort control (self-regulation) (Rothbart & Ahadi, 1994).

Thus, all children at birth would have an already inherited system for reactive responses of negative and positive affect and the biological basis of a system to control this reactivity. On Rothbart scales (Bosquet Enlow et al., 2016), negative affect items measure the tendency and intensity of negative emotional experiences, such as discomfort, fear or distress at novelty, anger and frustration, sadness, and low ability to remain calm. Extroversion/positive affect measures positive anticipatory response (curiosity and enthusiasm in the face of novel stimuli), high intensity pleasure, smiles and laughter, motor activity level, impulsivity, and degree of extroversion. Effort control measures attentional focus, inhibitory control, and low intensity pleasure (maintenance of pleasure when facing quieter and calmer activities).

It is interesting to note that, besides Rothbart, other authors have studied temperament and arrived at dimensions similar to those described to describe the constitutional differences studied in individuals (De Pauw & Mervielde, 2010). Thus, these dimensions that describe both emotional and behavioral reactivity and regulatory capacity seem to have consistency shown through different developmental theories.

Temperament: Adaptation and Psychopathology

The clinical importance of studying temperament lies in its relationship with mental health and psychopathology. Research shows that behaviors associated with different temperament components present from early development to later stages of childhood and adolescence, such as negative affect, extraversion/positive affect, and effort control, are related to both positive and socially accepted adaptations and "maladaptive" accommodations, i.e., behavioral adaptations seen as socially unacceptable or inappropriate (De Pauw & Mervielde, 2010).

Studies indicate that high levels of negative affect are associated with psychopathology (De Pauw & Mervielde, 2010). Throughout development, temperamental traits of intense emotional and motor reactivity of fear (more immediate response of alertness and vigilance, distress, and avoidance) and anxiety (slower response of apprehension and vigilance) are associated with symptoms of anxiety (including different diagnoses such as generalized and social anxiety), loneliness, low self-esteem, and depressive symptoms (De Pauw & Mervielde, 2010). Traits of intense emotional reactivity of sadness are associated with depressive symptoms at different ages of the child, while traits of intense reactivity of anger are associated with disruptive symptoms with associated diagnoses of aggressiveness and irritability (De Pauw & Mervielde, 2010). Temperament related to negative affect appears to be protected or exacerbated depending on individual self-regulation (De Pauw & Mervielde, 2010). For children with symptoms of anxiety or depression, the low attentional control capacity generates a difficulty in attentional shifting of sensations and feelings experienced, with potential exacerbation of symptoms. In other words, the low attentional capacity would be an aggravating factor of the negative emotional reactivity related to psychopathology.

Medium to high levels of extroversion and positive affect are associated with competence and social adaptation, although high levels of extroversion may be linked to psychopathology of impulsivity and potentially problematic social behaviors (De Pauw & Mervielde, 2010). On the other hand, significantly low extroversion traits, with low motor activity and little positive affect towards novel stimuli, are associated with depressive symptoms and dissatisfaction as well as anxiety and social isolation during different developmental stages (De Pauw & Mervielde, 2010).

Greater effort control with greater ability to perceive and direct attention and control reactive impulses is longitudinally related to adaptive behaviors in different contexts (Kochanska et al., 2010), whereas low regulatory capacity is associated with symptomatic behaviors such as inattention, impulsivity, and aggressiveness (Eisenberg et al., 2009), in addition to being an aggravating factor related to psychopathology. Low regulatory capacity may also be associated with pathological gambling and experience of social exclusion (Agrawal et al., 2012).

Although effort control is generally related to greater control of negative affect and greater well-being, when there is discrimination of the roles of "attention" and "inhibitory control" components, the findings may be paradoxical. For children with high rates of introversion, studies point out that high attentional levels could protect against anxious symptoms throughout development, while high inhibitory control would increase the risk for anxious symptoms (Moser et al., 2013). This paradox can be seen and explained by different studies that show that individuals with more fear and anxiety traits are more sensitive to control threats, being this exaggerated control a trigger to exacerbate anxious symptoms (Moser et al., 2013). This example shows the complexity of the interaction between subcomponents of reactivity and self-regulation, with multiple arrangements that can generate negative and positive outcomes.

Temperament and Parenting

The reciprocal interactions between parents and children are essential for the child's healthy development. One of the potential effects of these interactions is the caregiver's help in adjusting temperamental reactions and regulatory capacity with a greater chance of environmental child adaptation over time (Kiff et al., 2011). Thus, both temperament and parenting quality are distinct predictors of individual's adaptation.

For parenting to exert a healthy influence on temperamental characteristics, parents must primarily be sensitive to recognize and connect to their children's unique temperamental characteristics; the quality of this fit, called goodness-of-fit by researchers Thomas and Chess (1977), is a strong predictor of healthy psychological development. On the other hand, children's temperament generates parental emotional responses and consequently diverse behaviors, in a bidirectional and therefore transactional system, as already exposed in the chapter.

This bidirectional system can organize positive cycles (such as infant temperamental reactions that contribute to appropriate parental behaviors, which in turn adjust and shape the child's temperament in a positive way) or, on the other hand, negative cycles. Observing the dance between temperament and parental care, temperaments with greater vulnerability for psychopathology (as described in session above) also have greater susceptibility to suffer negative consequences in the face of inadequate parental care (Kiff et al., 2011). Children with more traits of negative affect (such as higher frustration intensity), impulsivity, and low effort control are more vulnerable to the adverse effects of inadequate parental care (such as negative monitoring, low affectivity, and strong intrusive control), while inadequate parental care may perpetuate or increase these described traits (Kiff et al., 2011). On the other hand, these same child temperamental characteristics are more likely to worsen the quality of parental care, precipitating or exacerbating intrusiveness, hostility, low affectivity, and parental neglect, in a negative bidirectional cycle (Kiff et al., 2011). Therefore, in clinical practice, it is essential to understand the biographical history linked to the child's temperamental characteristics, their effect and representation on parental care, and the quality and attunement of parenting to the specified child temperament of the observed child.

Conclusions

In this chapter, we describe, from a review of phylogenetic concepts and other fields of biology and developmental psychology, some aspects of the human organism that play a relevant role in determining its behaviors. We also emphasize the relevance of the reciprocal interactions between organism and environment in this process, including, as part of the environment in which the child develops, the parenting style exercised by its caregivers. The analysis of all these aspects is fundamental for a comprehensive and contextual clinical evaluation that takes into account the history of both individual biological characteristics and the interactions of these characteristics with the environment.

References

Agrawal, A., Verweij, K. J., Gillespie, N. A., Heath, A. C., Lessov-Schlaggar, C. N., Martin, N. G., Nelson, E. C., Slutske, W. S., Whitfield, J. B., & Lynskey, M. T. (2012). The genetics of addiction-a translational perspective. *Translational Psychiatry, 2*(7). https://doi.org/10.1038/tp.2012.54

Ayala, F. J. (2009). Darwin and the scientific method. *Proceedings of the National Academy of Sciences of the United States of America, 106*(1), 10033–10039. https://doi.org/10.1073/pnas.0901404106

Bani-Fatemi, A., Howe, A. S., & De Luca, V. (2015). Epigenetic studies of suicidal behavior. *Neurocase, 21*(2), 134–143. https://doi.org/10.1080/13554794.2013.826679

Bijou, S. (1993) Behavior analysis of child development context press edition in English - 2nd Rev.

Boero, F. (2015). From Darwin's origin of species toward a theory of natural history. *Prime Rep, 7*, 49. https://doi.org/10.12703/p7-49

Bosquet Enlow, M., White, M. T., Hails, K., Cabrera, I., & Wright, R. J. (2016). The infant behavior questionnaire-revised: Factor structure in a culturally and sociodemographically diverse sample in the United States. *Infant Behavior & Development, 43*, 24–35.

Burggren, W. W., & Crews, D. (2014). Epigenetics in comparative biology: Why we should pay attention. *Integrative and Comparative Biology, 54*(1), 7–20. https://doi.org/10.1093/icb/icu013

Burghardt, G. M. (2009). Darwin's legacy to comparative psychology and ethology. *The American Psychologist, 64*(2), 102–110. https://doi.org/10.1037/a0013385

Carlen, M. (2017). What constitutes the prefrontal cortex? *Science, 358*(6362), 478–482. https://doi.org/10.1126/science.aan8868

Carper, R. A., & Courchesne, E. (2005). Localized enlargement of the frontal cortex in early autism. *Biological Psychiatry, 57*(2), 126–133. https://doi.org/10.1016/j.biopsych.2004.11.005

Damasio, A., & Carvalho, G. B. (2013). The nature of feelings: Evolutionary and neurobiological origins. *Nature Reviews. Neuroscience, 14*(2), 143–152. https://doi.org/10.1038/nrn3403

De Pauw, S. S., & Mervielde, I. (2010). Temperament, personality and developmental psychopathology: A review based on the conceptual dimensions underlying childhood traits. *Child Psychiatry and Human Development, 41*(3), 313–329.

Decety, J., & Svetlova, M. (2012). Putting together phylogenetic and ontogenetic perspectives on empathy. *Developmental Cognitive Neuroscience, 2*(1), 1–24. https://doi.org/10.1016/j.dcn.2011.05.003

Deichmann, U. (2016). Epigenetics: The origins and evolution of a fashionable topic. *Developmental Biology, 416*(1), 249–254. https://doi.org/10.1016/j.ydbio.2016.06.005

Eisenberg, N., Chang, L., Ma, Y., & Huang, X. (2009). Relations of parenting style to Chinese children's effortful control, ego resilience, and maladjustment. *Development and Psychopathology, 21*(2), 455–477.

Emond, V., Joyal, C., & Poissant, H. (2009). Structural and functional neuroanatomy of attention-deficit hyperactivity disorder (ADHD). *Encephale, 35*(2), 107–114. https://doi.org/10.1016/j.encep.2008.01.005

Faraone, S. V., Asherson, P., Banaschewski, T., Biederman, J., Buitelaar, J. K., Ramos-Quiroga, J. A., & Franke, B. (2015). Attention-deficit/hyperactivity disorder. *Nature Reviews. Disease Primers, 1*, 15020. https://doi.org/10.1038/nrdp.2015.20

Fox, N. A., Henderson, H. A., Marshall, P. J., Nichols, K. E., & Ghera, M. M. (2005). Behavioral inhibition: Linking biology and behavior within a developmental framework. *Annual Review of Psychology, 56*, 235–262.

Fuster, J. M. (2001). The prefrontal cortex--an update: time is of the essence. In: Neuron 30, 319–333.

Fuster, J. M. (2002). Frontal lobe and cognitive development. Journal of Neurocytology, 31(3–5), 373–385.

Gonzalez-Pardo, H., & Perez Alvarez, M. (2013). Epigenetics and its implications for psychology. *Psicothema, 25*(1), 3–12. https://doi.org/10.7334/psicothema2012.327

Hess, U., & Thibault, P. (2009). Darwin and emotion expression. *The American Psychologist, 64*(2), 120–128. https://doi.org/10.1037/a0013386

Hsu, N. S., & Jaeggi, S. M. (2014). The emergence of cognitive control abilities in childhood. *Current Topics in Behavioral Neurosciences, 16*, 149–166. https://doi.org/10.1007/7854_2013_241

Kiff, C. J., Lengua, L. J., & Zalewski, M. (2011). Nature and nurturing: Parenting in the context of child temperament. *Clinical Child and Family Psychology Review, 14*(3), 251–301.

Kochanska, G., Koenig, J. L., Barry, R. A., Kim, S., & Yoon, J. E. (2010). Children's conscience during toddler and preschool years, moral self, and a competent, adaptive developmental trajectory. *Developmental Psychology, 46*(5), 1320–1332.

Miller, E. K. (2000). The prefrontal cortex and cognitive control. *Nature Reviews. Neuroscience, 1*(1), 59–65. https://doi.org/10.1038/35036228

Moser, J. S., Moran, T. P., Schroder, H. S., Donnellan, M. B., & Yeung, N. (2013). On the relationship between anxiety and error monitoring: A meta-analysis and conceptual framework. *Frontiers in Human Neuroscience, 7*, 466.

Nigg, J. T. (2016). Where do epigenetics and developmental origins take the field of developmental psychopathology? *Journal of Abnormal Child Psychology, 44*(3), 405–419. https://doi.org/10.1007/s10802-015-0121-9

Posner, M. I., & Rothbart, M. K. (1998). Attention, self-regulation and consciousness. *Philosophical Transactions of the Royal Society of London. Series B, Biological Sciences, 353*(1377), 1915–1927.

Rothbart, M. K., & Ahadi, S. A. (1994). Temperament and the development of personality. *Journal of Abnormal Psychology, 103*, 55–66.

Rothbart, M. K., Ahadi, S. A., Hershey, K. L., & Fisher, P. (2001). Investigations of temperament at three to seven years: The Children's behavior questionnaire. *Child Development, 72*(5), 1394–1408.

Sameroff, A. J. (2009). The transactional model. In A. Sameroff (Ed.), *The transactional model of development: How children and contexts shape each other* (pp. 3–21).

Sameroff, A. J., & MacKenzie, M. J. (2003). A quarter-century of the transactional model: How have things changed? *Zero to Three, 24*(1), 9.

Shaw, P., Eckstrand, K., Sharp, W., Blumenthal, J., Lerch, J. P., Greenstein, D., & Rapoport, J. L. (2007). Attention-deficit/hyperactivity disorder is characterized by a delay in cortical maturation. *Proceedings of the National Academy of Sciences of the United States of America, 104*(49), 19649–19654. https://doi.org/10.1073/pnas.0707741104

Teffer, K., & Semendeferi, K. (2012). Human prefrontal cortex: Evolution, development, and pathology. *Progress in Brain Research*, 195. Elsevier.

Thomas, A., & Chess, S. (1977). *Temperament and development*. Brunner/Mazel.

Thomas, A., Chess, S., Birch, H. G., Hertzig, M. E., & Korn, S. (1963). *Behavioral individuality in early childhood*. New York University.

Weaver, I. C., Cervoni, N., Champagne, F. A., D'Alessio, A. C., Sharma, S., Seckl, J. R., & Meaney, M. J. (2004). Epigenetic programming by maternal behavior. *Nature Neuroscience, 7*(8), 847–854. https://doi.org/10.1038/nn1276

Chapter 5
Clinical Assessment in Clinical Behavior Analysis for Children and Definition of Therapeutic Goals

Ila Marques Porto Linares , Adriana Suzart Ungaretti Rossi ,
Maíra P. Toscano, and Verena L. Hermann

As described in previous chapters of this book, child intervention from an behavior analysis' perspective is composed of different stages, including the initial assessment, which aims to collect data through interviews with parents and professionals involved, as well as through assessment sessions of the child's behavior. This evaluation seeks to gather the largest amount of information in order to help the therapist in the formulation of the case and intervention. Thus, the more information collected at this stage of clinical care, the broader the understanding of the case and the greater the chance of formulating complete functional analyses.

The conduct of the initial assessment may take several paths, to be chosen by the clinical behavior analyst. The literature in the area presents different positions on what the initial assessment (or diagnostic assessment) encompasses. After a non-systematic bibliographic survey, no consolidated model was found to perform this relevant stage of child care. Among the models in the literature, for example, Silvares (2000) proposes that the diagnostic assessment comprises four phases, namely, (1) identification of problems, concluding their nature and possibility of treatment, (2) functional analysis, (3) treatment selection, and (4) treatment evaluation. In turn, for Kanfer and Saslow (1976), the assessment comprises seven steps: (1) initial assessment of the problem situation, (2) clarification of the problem situation, (3) motivational analysis, (4) developmental analysis, (5) self-control

---

I. M. P. Linares
Universidade de São Paulo, São Paulo, Brazil
e-mail: ila.linares@hc.fm.usp.br

A. S. U. Rossi
Paradigma – Center for Behavioral Sciences and Technology, São Paulo, Brazil
e-mail: adrianarossi@paradigmaac.org

M. P. Toscano · V. L. Hermann (✉)
Private Practice, São Paulo, Brazil
e-mail: mairatoscano@gmail.com; verenalhermann@gmail.com

© The Author(s), under exclusive license to Springer Nature Switzerland AG 2022
A. S. U. Rossi et al. (eds.), *Clinical Behavior Analysis for Children*,
https://doi.org/10.1007/978-3-031-12247-7_5

analysis, (6) analysis of social relationships, and (7) analysis of the socio-physical-cultural environment.

Regra (2012) describes in detail each step of the initial assessment and makes the following division: (1) data survey with description of the undesirable behaviors; (2) survey of hypotheses that may be favoring the occurrence of the target behaviors; (3) survey of the most likely hypotheses about the variables that may be hindering the occurrence of the desirable behaviors; (4) presentation of the work proposal; (5) initial guidance of selected simple situations, to expedite the process of change; and (6) closing of the therapeutic contract.

In Naves and Ávila's (2018) text on case formulation, the behavioral assessment requires the therapist to consider behavioral patterns and functional relationships established in the child's current and past history. Investigations regarding client data; child development; life, family, academic, medical, and psychological histories; as well as therapeutic routine and goals are the main steps that make up the assessment in case formulation.

From theory to practice, there seem to be different positions on the form of assessment to be developed in the clinic by the child behavior analyst. Del Prette et al. (2005) assessed 20 Brazilian studies of clinical behavior analysis for children and concluded that, in general, initial assessments with parents and child, as well as interviews with parents during therapy, predominate. As for the method of data collection, the main one is the observation in session, before, during, and after the interventions (without reference to systematic record). In addition, in less than half of the cases, there was reapplication of instruments initially applied or of assessment at the end.

Still referring to the way the initial assessment is conducted, some authors highlight the relevance of using different playful strategies (e.g., drawings and make-believe games) that facilitate the therapist's access to relevant information. This is because, in general, children are not always able to accurately report daily events. Thus, in addition to accessing information by observing the child's behavioral patterns while playing, the clinician can also collect data on the daily life through questions during play (Del Prette & Meyer, 2012; Del Rey, 2012).

The difference between the stages of assessment and intervention is not a consensus in the area. Bertolla and Brandão (2017), for example, argue that assessment and intervention are not formally differentiated in the literature and, in practice, both take place simultaneously throughout the therapeutic process. Thus, there is not a set number of sessions for this initial period of information collection. In all stages of the progress of the case, the therapist gathers information that may be relevant to the functional analysis.

Converging with the abovementioned authors, Conte and Regra (2012) state that, from the initial contact with the family, data are collected and interventions possibly leading to changes are implemented. Thus, it is not characterized a moment of assessment and another of intervention throughout the child care. For them, these moments happen intertwined during the sessions.

The authors who advocate the non-differentiation between assessment and intervention explain that waiting for the completion of an assessment to then start the intervention becomes unfeasible, given the urgency required by many cases. There are also situations in which a complete assessment is not always necessary for the intervention to take place (Conte & Regra, 2012). In these situations, intervention and assessment go hand in hand.

Despite the distinct positions between the moments of assessment and intervention, it is understood that the structuring of the stages of an initial therapeutic assessment, with defined phases and specific objectives, can be of great use for the therapist and for the family who seeks therapy. For the therapist, a good clinical practice requires the ability to gather data to build consistent functional analyses and to define therapeutic objectives. For the family, this structuring facilitates the understanding that there is an outline to be followed during the work, also combating possible myths that the therapeutic process would be unstructured.

Finally, it is clear that there are several difficulties faced in the evaluation process and, more specifically, in the delimitation of an initial evaluation moment, given the breadth of possibilities. In order to systematize and contribute to the construction of the evaluation process in the clinical behavior analysis for children, a material prepared by the authors of this chapter will be presented, consisting of different elements that are described in the literature of the area.

Proposal for Evaluation

Based on some needs observed by the authors during the initial assessment process, a critical analysis of the literature already produced so far was conducted, leading to the proposition of an initial assessment framework.

As a fruit of this work, the proposed initial evaluation framework lasts 5 to 7 weeks and consists of the following steps:

1. Initial interview and therapeutic contract.
2. Application of complementary instruments.
3. Child observation.
4. Assessment of child-caregiver interaction.
5. Contact with school and other professionals.
6. Feedback to parents.

Below is a brief description of each of the steps that make up this process.

Initial Interview and Therapeutic Contract

The initial interview is conducted with parents (or caregivers) and lasts from one to two sessions. In line with the model proposed by Regra (2012), the initial interview with parents can be divided into a unstructured interview – when parents freely report their concerns – and, subsequently, a structured interview, in which the therapist asks questions to guide the parents' discourse, thus helping professionals build a functional analysis.

The questions asked by the therapist aim to investigate aspects related to the main complaint and the contexts in which it manifests itself, i.e., possible antecedent and consequent variables that may be contributing to the maintenance of the problem behavior (Vermes, 2012). It also seeks to investigate aspects of the child's environment, such as the educational practices adopted by parents, family structure and dynamics, relationships with peers, educational performance, etc. At this time, possible reinforcing stimuli for the child are also investigated to assist in planning the initial sessions with the child.

It is essential that the therapist considers that the reports brought depend on the parents' capacity of observation and description and are often a cutout of the behavior. Thus, environmental variables that may be contributing to the maintenance of the problem are not always described. Thus, it is up to the therapist to select relevant information from the report in order to build functional analyses.

After gathering this data, a summary is made for the parents of the main points that were discussed, and, whenever possible, initial orientations are also offered in relation to some of the problems presented. Such orientations, although certainly not covering all the possible solutions to the complaints presented, may offer relief to the most immediate difficulties. In addition to having the purpose of producing small changes in the environment, they may contribute to the engagement of parents in the therapeutic process. Next, the theoretical approach from which the therapeutic process will be conducted is presented, as well as the structure of the assessment to be performed with the child and parents.

It is worth remembering that, still in the initial session, it is verified if the parents have already discussed with the child the beginning of the therapeutic work. If this has not yet occurred, guidance is offered on ways to do so. For example, the parents may tell the child that he will start seeing a psychologist, who is someone who studies feelings and behavior, and that this professional will help him better understand what he feels, as well as receive help to better deal with what is happening. Then, with the psychologist, he will talk, play, draw, and do various activities (Vermes, 2012). Alternatively, it is possible to suggest that parents make a parallel between the therapist and another professional by whom the child has already been seen (e.g., psychiatrist or pediatrician), relating the psychologist to someone who works together with the professional with whom they already have some kind of bond established. In this same context, Bertolla and Brandão (2017) suggest telling the child that he/she will meet a friend of the psychiatrist, doctor, or other professional who made the referral. It is worth pointing out that each therapist will gradually find his own way of presenting his work to the child and may, of course, present himself in different ways, considering the particularities of each case.

Finally, it is important that the therapeutic contract is established, covering issues related to the format of the work. At this moment, therefore, agreements are made about the duration and frequency of sessions, absences, delays, joint and individual sessions, how the contact by phone is made, payment, vacations, orientation session and parent training, and family session, among others (cf. Regra, 2012).

Application of Complementary Instruments

The initial interview is a moment when parents usually feel distressed about the difficulties they are experiencing and are sometimes anxious to meet the professional who will conduct the work. In this stage of the process, the therapist, in addition to listening and welcoming the parents, also has a series of other objectives, such as those discussed in step 1. In practical terms, these are objectives that require considerable time, and, in this context, it is very useful to use other means to complement the investigation.

Data collection can also occur through the completion of supplementary materials, questionnaires, or inventories delivered to parents as a way to investigate important information. Such documents can be filled out by parents in between sessions and aim to investigate areas related to the child's behavior, parenting practices, and the main caregiver's mood, for example.

Evidently, it is up to the therapist to evaluate which material or instrument best suits the case and the data they seek to know. However, for the investigation of data on clinical history, psychosocial and health aspects, school life, routine, and family, among others, the delivery of the Initial Assessment form (Annex I) is suggested. In addition, some other questionnaires and materials related to areas of investigation recurrently present in the child's clinic are recommended, which can be useful for the collection of complementary data.

Registration form – particular to each professional.
Routine description – material for filling in the activities of the child's routine.
Inventory or questionnaire screening for child problem behaviors. Example: Child Behavior Checklist (CBCL) (Achenbach, 1991; Bordin et al., 1995).
Frequency map of problem behaviors (Regra, 2012) – document for recording situations referring to the complaint and the times when they occur.
Questionnaire/assessment developed by the therapist to investigate autonomy in relation to activities of daily living – when pertinent.
Questionnaire for the investigation of the main caregivers' mood. Example: Beck Depression Inventory (BDI-II) (Gorenstein et al., 2011).
Questionnaire for research on parenting practices.
Questionnaire for collecting data on the child's behavior at school.

Observation of the Child

For this stage, two sessions with the child are planned, which have, as one of their main objectives, the beginning of the establishment of the therapeutic bond (Regra, 2012). Other objectives include building, together with the child, an understanding of what the therapeutic process is and how it takes place, presenting confidentiality as an element of the therapeutic relationship, establishing agreements in relation to the sessions' structures, and conducting observation, which will allow for the identification of target behaviors for intervention and the child's general repertoire (Vermes, 2012).

To identify target behaviors, playful activities and games appropriate to the client's age are used. Through these resources, we seek to produce antecedent stimuli that evoke responses from the child associated with the clinically relevants behaviors. It is understood that the emission of clinically relevant behaviors during the session allows the therapist to observe responses that will potentially be targets of intervention, as well as important data for the construction of the functional analysis and the establishment of a baseline for the intervention.

During the initial sessions with the child, aspects related to compliance with rules and sociability with the interlocutor, among other skills, are also observed, with the objective of evaluating the child's total repertoire. We seek to identify behavioral deficits and excesses, as well as desirable responses already installed, which may become important resources in the development of alternative responses to problem situations or even serve as intermediate responses to be reinforced in a modeling process.

In this stage of the evaluation, the "Support material for the child therapist" (Annex II) is suggested as support material for the therapist, which offers a description of items to be evaluated during contact with the child. This material guides the therapist's observation, directing the recording of several classes of responses that, in general, are important in a child's repertoire. It becomes an antecedent stimulus for the therapist to reflect on the stage of development of various abilities of the child.

Through this material, the following items are investigated: identification of possible reinforcers, rule-following, self-knowledge, frustration, self-control and emotional expressiveness, civility, empathy, assertiveness, problem-solving, and academic skills. This material also includes the record therapist's mediation for the items in which the child does not demonstrate autonomy of execution. Thus, it is evaluated and recorded whether, with a certain level of help, the child would be able to perform the investigated behavior.

Thus, based on the child's observation sessions, the therapist will build a kind of panorama regarding the child's current difficulties and potential, which will serve as a baseline for the target behaviors. This baseline will be followed throughout the therapeutic process in order to assess the impact of the intervention and possible progress in the child's behavior.

Assessment of Child-Caregiver Interaction

At this moment of the assessment, activities are proposed with the objective of evaluating the dynamics of interaction of the child with the primary caregiver. Since the individual's behavior varies according to the context and the reinforcement scheme in place, it is relevant to observe how the child behaves in the presence of his parents. As part of the variables that will determine the emission and maintenance of certain behaviors, it is especially important to observe how parents react to some behaviors. That is, through child-parent interactions, one seeks information on how parents deal with the child's difficulties, that is, whether they exercise some form of punishment or help the child to develop the repertoire for the emission of an appropriate response. With the same degree of relevance, the parents' reaction to the child's appropriate behaviors is observed, that is, if they offer some form of description and appreciation or if they present some consequence in order to increase the probability of future occurrence of such classes of responses.

The second part of the "Supporting material for the child therapist" (Annex II) is proposed to be used to record the data obtained in relation to the parents, which can also contribute to the collection of relevant data for the formulation of the case. The data can be obtained (1) through the parents' report and observation of the child, (2) through observation during the child's session with the parents, and (3) through contacts with the parents in the waiting room and scheduling situations. The items of this support material are related to the following aspects: parenting practices, parents' social skills, family, parental motivation, and concerns.

Contact with School and Other Professionals

After the previous steps, it is suggested to establish contact with the school and other professionals who accompany the child. In the contact with the school, general perceptions of the teachers and coordinators regarding the child are investigated, both in relation to the concerns brought by the parents and to general aspects of the child's behavior, including student attitude, academic performance, and socialization. Also in the "Support material for the child therapist" (Annex II), there is a specific section about expected behaviors in the classroom context and in the relationship with peers and teachers, which can serve as guidance for the therapist. More specifically regarding problem behaviors, it is important to ask how these responses occur in the school context, investigating antecedent and consequent stimuli that may be contributing to their maintenance.

Sometimes the school's report on the child's problem-behavior may be different from the family's report. This difference, among other factors, may be related to behavioral changes that may occur according to variations in the environments in which the child is inserted. This is important data for the therapist to evaluate environmental specificities favorable to the appearance of the complaint. When pertinent, it is possible to offer guidance to professionals who work with the child at school, in order to favor the initial management of the problem issues.

In addition, it is valid to establish what will be the best channel of communication between professionals (e.g., email and/or telephone), so that the exchange of information and guidance can occur continuously, as needed. In addition, the need for contact with other professionals who accompany the child, such as learning specialist, speech therapist, occupational therapist, psychiatrist, and neuropediatrician, among others, is reinforced. Such contact can help the professional to gather important data on the history and also allows an aligned performance among professionals, offering an interdisciplinary approach.

Feedback to Parents

With all the data collected in the previous steps and through the analysis of the complementary instruments, the therapist should develop the case formulation. This process includes functionally analyzing the complaint-behavior, establishing the target behavior(s) of the intervention, and defining the form of action (cf. Eells, 2007).

For the feedback session, only the presence of the caregivers is required. Feedback is given on the clinical observations, the initial hypotheses, the initial intervention plan, and the structure of the work to be performed. Next, the aspects that the therapist believes should also be the target of the intervention should be presented. It is worth noting that not always what is put forward by the parents as a complaint covers what the therapist observed as clinical demand during the evaluation process. Thus, it is recommended that in the feedback session the therapeutic objectives be aligned with those of the parents so that they can adjust their expectations in relation to the therapeutic work. In this way, parents can also actively participate in the intervention, increasing engagement and therefore the possibility of successful therapy. Objectives are usually related to aspects that should be managed throughout the therapeutic process, both in relation to the child's repertoire and to the manipulation of environmental variables. Such objectives must obey a priority criterion, since covering all issues at the same time may cause the intervention to lack the solidity required for change. Therefore, the relevance of a given objective should be verified at each moment of the progress of the case, as well as the possibility of reaching the goal and the intermediate steps necessary for the long-term objectives to be achieved (Eells, 2007).

Regarding the structure of the work to be done, each case has its own particularities. In some cases, the intervention occurs more directly with the child. For example, one may aim to develop repertoires of naming feelings and ability to tolerate discomfort, which will allow the child to be more successful in dealing with the challenges posed by the environment. In other cases, a more intense parental participation may be crucial for the clinical intervention to allow the rearrangement of environmental contingencies through parental guidance and/or training or family sessions. Many times, the active participation of school professionals is also requested, as they constitute an important part of the child's environment.

The request for parents' participation, either more distantly or more closely, often faces some barriers. Some parents are unwilling to engage directly in the therapeutic process, justified by lack of time, low motivation to review their parenting practices, or by the expectation that the issue will be solved without the family's involvement. When these and other difficulties are observed, it is important that the parental motivation to participate in therapy is investigated and that the need for the parents' active partnership is clarified for the development of the work.

In addition to the points raised, the need for periodic monitoring of therapeutic objectives both for verification of the effectiveness of the process and for the establishment of the following objectives is also emphasized. That is, despite the information obtained and the objectives outlined in the initial assessment, it is understood that the assessment process needs to be maintained throughout the psychotherapeutic care. Additionally, it is understood that the verification of the effectiveness of the process should be composed by the report of the parents, the child, and other people of the acquaintanceship, as well as by the clinical observation of the therapist in session.

Conclusion

This chapter aimed to present a proposal for an initial structured assessment that includes an interview with the parents, observation of the child and of parental practices, and contact with the school and other professionals involved in the case. A proper delineation of the case may contribute to more targeted and effective interventions, increasing the likelihood of success in therapeutic intervention. Finally, it is worth pointing out that this is a specific proposal for a comprehensive topic, which is not restricted to a single model. Thus, it is expected that a continuous improvement of this model will occur.

Annex-I

INITIAL ASSESSMENT FORM

IDENTIFICATION	
Date:	
Patient's name:	
Age:	Date of birth:
Questionnaire completed by:	
Address:	

Neighborhood: City: ZIP CODE:

Home phone:

With whom does the patient reside?

....

Mother's name:

Training:	Occupation:

Mother's contact phone number:

Father's name:

Training:	Occupation:

Father's contact phone number:

Name and age of siblings:

....

School name:

Coordinator:	Professor:
Year:	Class:

Other professionals accompanying the case (name, profession and contact telephone number):

....

ISSUE
Reason for seeking therapy (describe):

....

ANALYSIS

How and how long ago did the problem appear?
....
....
....
....

Cite which contexts increase the problem:
....
....
....
....

Name the contexts in which the problem does not appear or appears less frequently:
....
....
....
....
....

How does the family currently deal with the child at times when the problem manifests itself?
....
....
....
....
....

CLINICAL HISTORY

PREGNANCY

Planned pregnancy: ( ) yes ( ) no

Complications (in pregnancy or delivery): ( ) yes ( ) no

Id:
....
....
....

Use of substance: ( ) yes ( ) no

Specify which and the frequency of use:
....
....
....

HEALTH CHANGES	Any change in health: ( ) yes ( ) no ( ) do not know Id: .... Any developmental delay? ( ) yes ( ) no ( ) I do not know Id: .... Hospitalization for diseases or accidents? ( ) yes ( ) no ( ) I do not know What happened and when it happened: .... Have you ever had neuropsychological evaluation? ( ) yes ( ) no When: ....
NEUROPSYCHOMOTOR DEVELOPMENT	Age when he walked without support: .... Age when he spoke his first words: .... Age of defrosting: -Daytime: -Evening: ....

PSYCHOSOCIAL AND HEALTH ASPECTS	
	Stressful events prior to the current symptoms: ( ) yes ( ) no Id: .... Important changes in life: ( ) yes ( ) no Id: .... How was the family's life at the time of the onset of the difficulties? Changes: ....

Financial situation:

Marital difficulties:

Difficulties with other children or family members:

PSYCHOSOCIAL AND HEALTH CONDITIONS

Diseases:

Diagnoses and comorbidities: ( ) yes ( ) no

Identify (note age at onset):

Use of regular medications? ( ) yes ( ) no

Name, dosage and time of administration:

Follow-up with other health professionals: ( ) yes ( ) no

Specify:

Cognitive development (compared to peers):

( ) equivalent ( ) above ( ) below

Specify:

Emotional development (purchased in pairs):

( ) equivalent ( ) above ( ) below

Specify:

When faced with new or stressful situations, he tends to have a posture: ( ) withdrawn ( ) exploratory

Self-regulation in the face of stressful situations (from preschool to the present):

Perceived skills, abilities and potentials (list and describe):
....
....
....
....
....

Relationship with peers (from preschool to the present):
....
....
....
....
....
....
....

Acceptance among peers: ( )high ( )medium ( )low
Specify:
....

PEER RELATIONSHIPS

Make friends easily? ( ) yes ( ) no

What are the name of his closest friends?
....
....
....
....

Have you ever been a victim of *bullying*, including *cyberbullying*: ( ) yes ( ) no

What happened:
....
....
....

SCHOOL LIFE

Age of school entry:

Adjustment to school start (describe):
....
....
....
....

SCHOOL LIFE

Which schools has he studied?
....
....

Name of the school	*Period*
....	
....	
....	
....	

Reason for exchange(s):
....
....

Child's current school experience:
- School schedule: ....
- Period: ....
- Academic performance (compared to peers): ( )equivalent ( )above ( )below

Specify: ....
- School support - Does the school support and collaborate with family positions and requests? ( ) yes ( )no
Describe: ....
....

Extracurricular activities: ( ) yes ( ) no
Identify (note frequency and when they occur): ....
....

Participation of the child in other out-of-school groups: ( ) yes ( ) no
Id: ....

ROUTINE

What is the child's study routine like at home?
....
....

Does the child do his homework on his own or with others?
....
....

STUDY ROUTINE	Does the child have free time to play? At what times? ....
	Does the child help with household chores? Which ones? ....
FOOD ROUTINE	Eating routine (describe time and what is consumed): ....
	The times of meals are regular? ( ) yes ( ) no
	Does he accept well a variety of foods or are there any restrictions? Explain: ....
	Are meals taken at the table? ( ) yes ( ) no If yes, does the child remain at the table until the end of the meal? ( ) yes ( ) no
	Are meals taken separately or together with others? ( ) separate ( ) joint
	Does the child use any device (mobile phone, TV, tablet) during the meal? ( ) yes ( ) no Which ones: ....
SLEEP ROUTINE	- Usual bedtime:
	- Usual time to wake up:
	- Does the child take naps during the day? How many and at what time? ....
	- Does the child have pre-sleep routine? ( ) yes ( )no
EXERCISE ROUTINE	- Type and frequency of exercise: ....

	FAMILY
MEMBERS	Siblings: ( ) yes ( ) no Name and age: ....
FAMILY HISTORY	History of mental illness in the family: ( ) yes ( ) no Which (note the relationship): ....
RELATIONSHIPS	Long-lasting separations from those responsible: ( ) yes ( ) no Running time: Relationship between mother and child: ( ) assertive ( ) passive ( ) aggressive Describe: Relationship between parent and child: ( ) assertive ( ) passive ( ) aggressive Describe: Relationship between siblings and child:( ) assertive ( ) passive ( ) aggressive Describe: Handling done in situations of conflict with siblings (describe): Other family conflicts (list the main ones): .... Do you carry out activities together? Which ones? ....

	Family identification with some cultural or religious tradition: ( ) yes ( ) no .... Specify: ....
CULTURAL/RELIGIOUS ASPECTS	Cultural/religious practices: ( ) yes ( ) no Which ones: ....

FINAL ASSESSMENT	
FINAL ASSESSMENT	How do you understand/explain the difficulties that the child currently presents? .... Describe: .... Is the child aware of his/her own difficulty? .... Describe: ....

Annex-II

Support material for the child therapist

Items to direct observation in session with the child		Does	Does with mediation	Does not	OBS
Survey of reinforceers	Appropriately describes preferred activities				
	Describes preferred foods				
	Names friends, family activities, tv shows, games, preferred sports				
Following rules	Accepts to interrupt ongoing activities during the waiting time at the reception				
	Respects the proposed session format				
	Follows the rules of activities and games				
	Accepts when prompted about session termination				
	In fantasy activities, demonstrates knowledge of social rules				
Self-knowledge	Appropriately speaks of lived experiences (those heard, felt, seen, and thought about)				
	Describes your behavior patterns				
	Orally describes contingencies related to the complaint				
	Describes contingencies of your life through playful resources				
	Describes characteristics that you consider qualities				
	Describes characteristics that you consider difficulties/defects				
	Describes characteristics that you consider important to develop/work				
	Can understand the relationship between experienced events and their emotions				
Frustration	Accepts when you are denied something you ask/would like to do				
	Asks for help/persists when he/she perceives difficulty in performing some activity				
	When he loses, he seeks alternative answers to achieve the proposed goal (asks for rematch, tries in other ways, etc.)				
	Shows proper competitiveness during the game				
	Has a regulated emotional response when losing in the game				

Support material for the child therapist					
Self-control and emotional expressivity	Knows how to name their own emotions and those of others				
	Can you describe your feelings in situations experienced				
	Tolerates frustrations				
	Demonstrates appropriate anger management				
	Demonstrates proper voice modulation				
	Expresses other emotions (e.g., fear/joy/sadness) appropriately				
Civility	Greets and says goodbye properly				
	Uses expressions of gratitude				
	Waits for your turn to speak				
	Asks and answers questions				
	Gives and accepts compliments				
	Respects hierarchy				
	Calls the interlocutor by name or nickname (e.g., aunt)				
Empathy	Shows interest in others				
	Observes				
	Pays attention to each other				
	Demonstrates listening to the other, responding to requests				
	Shows interest in others				
	Infers feelings from the interlocutor and demonstrates putting himself in their place				
	Expresses understanding of the other's feelings				
	Shows respect for differences				
	Offers help				
	Shares something you have				
Assertivity	Expresses negative feelings				
	Talks about strengths and weaknesses (of the other and of oneself)				
	Can maintain a dialogue initiated by the interlocutor				
	Agrees and disagrees opinions				
	Makes and declines orders				
	Deals with criticism and mockery				
	Asks for behavior change				
	Negotiates conflicting interests				
	Defends your own rights				
	Resists peer pressure				

Support material for the child therapist					
Problem-solving	Remains calm in the face of a problem situation				
	Recognizes and names different types of problems				
	Thinks before making decisions				
	Identifies and evaluates possible solution alternatives, chooses				
	Chooses, implements, and evaluates an alternative				
	Evaluates the decision-making process				
Academic skills	Follows rules or oral instructions				
	Observes and pays attention to what is said				
	Ignores peer interruptions				
	Imitates socially competent behaviors				
	Waits for your turn to speak				
	Asks and answers questions				
	Offers, requests, and appreciates help				
	Seeks approval for performance performed				
	Praises and appreciates compliments				
	Recognizes the quality of the other's performance				
	Fulfills orders				
	Cooperates and participates in discussions				

Items to direct observation of the environments in which the child is part		Observed data
Parenting practices	What disciplinary techniques do or do not work well?	
	Parents converge in parenting opinions and practices	
	What is the child's reaction to the parents' practices?	
	Quality of the commands (topography and what is produced with the commands)***	
	Parents are effective in describing and valuing desirable behaviors	
	Physical abuse	
	Inconsistent punishment (parents punish or reinforce the child's behaviors non-contingently)	
	Relaxed discipline (non-compliance with rules set by parents)	
	Negative monitoring (excessive supervision / large number of repetitive instructions)	
	Neglect (not attentive to the needs of their children)	
	Positive monitoring (parents' attention and knowledge about where their child is and the activities carried out)	
	Moral behavior (transmit values)	
	Parents demonstrate self-knowledge about the parenting practices used	
Social skills of parents	Follow parents' rules	
	Reaction to frustration (in the relationship with the child)	
	Self-control and emotional expressiveness	
	Civility	
	Show empathy with the child	
	Assertiveness when expressing yourself	

Items to direct observation of the environments in which the child is part		Observed data
Family	Relationship with siblings	
	Mediation made by parents in the relationship between children	
	Relationship with mother	
	Relationship with father	
	Relationship between parents	
	Relationship with another caregiver	
	Family dynamics	
	Parents' report on compliance with ADLs	
	Does it help with household chores?	
	Who gives more attention to the child? Why?	
	Do you spend a lot of time away from your parents?	
	Who in the family group does the child most identify with? Why? What are the identification points?	
Parental motivation	Parents understand that solving the problem will also depend on changes in their own behavior.	
	Parents are available to attend treatment	
	Parents are available to be involved in treatment (albeit remotely)	
	Parents are willing to learn and apply the guidelines given in the session at home	
	Parents are willing to review their parenting practices to help their child	
Complaint	What are the attempts made by the parents to resolve the complaint and what are the results obtained?	
	How did the complaint evolve, was there a change in frequency and intensity?	
	What are people's current reactions to complaint behaviors and why?	
	Does the child agree or disagree with the parent's complaint?	
School	Academic achievement	
	Relationship with peers	
	Is the school aware of the complaint?	
	Child self-regulation at school	
	Any school adaptation for the child?	
	Child's relationship with teachers	

Items to direct observation of the environments in which the child is part		Observed data
Friends	Do you make friends easily?	
	Who are the child's friends?	
	Is it very requested by the group of friends?	
	How are the relationships with colleagues, neighbors, etc.?	
Relevant data from the questionnaire		

References

Achenbach, T. M. (1991). *Manual for the child behavior checklist/4–18*. University of Vermont, Department of Psychiatry.

Bertolla, M. H. S. M., & Brandão, L. C. (2017). *Orientações para psicoterapeutas infantis iniciantes* (Desenvolvimento de material didático ou instrucional – Manual).

Bordin, I. S., Mari, J., & Caeiro, M. F. (1995). Validação da versão brasileira do child behavior checklist – inventário de comportamentos da infância e adolescência: dados preliminares. *Revista Brasileira Psiquiatria, 17*(2), 55–66.

Conte, F. C. S., & Regra, J. A. G. (2012). A psicoterapia comportamental infantil: novos aspectos. In Silvares, E. F. M. (Ed.), *Estudos de caso em psicologia clínica comportamental infantil*. Papirus Editora.

Silvares, E. F. M (2000). Avaliação e intervenção clínica comportamental infantil. In: Silvares, E. F. M. (Ed.), *Estudos de caso em psicologia clínica comportamental infantil* (Vol. 1, pp. 13–30). Papirus Editora.

Del Prette, G., & Meyer, S. B. (2012). O brincar como ferramenta de avaliação e intervenção. Em N. B. Borges & F. A. Cassas (Orgs.), *Clínica analítico-comportamental: Aspectos teóricos e práticos*. Artmed.

Del Prette, G., de Silvares, E. F. M., & Meyer, S. B. (2005). Validade interna em 20 estudos de caso comportamentais brasileiros sobre terapia infantil. *Revista Brasileira de Terapia Comportamental e Cognitiva, 12*(1), 93–105.

Del Rey, D. (2012). O uso de recursos lúdicos na avaliação funcional em clínica analítico-comportamental infantil. Em N. B. Borges & F. A. Cassas (Orgs.), *Clínica analítico-comportamental: Aspectos teóricos e práticos*. Artmed.

Eells, T. D. (2007). *Handbook of psychotherapy case formulation* (2nd ed.). The Guilford Press.

Gorenstein, C., Pang, W. Y., Argimon, I. L., & Werlang, B. S. G. (2011). *Inventário Beck de Depressão-II*. Manual. Casa do Psicólogo.

Kanfer, F. H., & Saslow, G. (1976). An outline for behavioral diagnosis. In E. E. J. Mash & L. G. Terdal (Eds.), *Behavioral therapy assessment* (cap. 5). Springer.

Naves, A. R. C. X., & Ávila, A. R. R. (2018). A formulação comportamental na terapia analítico-comportamental infantil. In: A. K. C. R. Em De-Farias, F. N. Fonseca, & L. B. Nery (Orgs.), *Teoria e formulação de casos em análise comportamental clínica* (pp. 185–213). Artmed.

Regra, J. A. G. (2012). As entrevistas iniciais na clínica analítico-comportamental infantil. In: Em N. B. Borges, & F. A. Cassas (Orgs.), *Clínica analítico-comportamental: Aspectos teóricos e práticos* (pp. 185–213). Artmed.

Vermes, J. S. (2012). Clínica analítico-comportamental infantil: a estrutura. In: N. Em Borges, & F. A. Cassas, *Clínica analítico-comportamental: aspectos teóricos e práticos* (pp. 214–222). Artmed.

Chapter 6
Evidence-Based Psychotherapy in Childhood and Adolescence

Jan Luiz Leonardi and José Luiz Dias Siqueira

In the early 1990s, a task force of Division 12 of the *American Psychological Association* (Society for Clinical Psychology) developed a set of criteria to establish a psychological intervention as an "empirically sustained treatment" (Chambless, 1993). This required that it meet two criteria: (1) it had to be described in a manual, to standardize procedures (the independent variable in question), and thus enable therapists to replicate what had been previously tested, and (2) there had to be experimental evidence proving its efficacy, which could come from two or more randomized clinical trials or from a set of single-case experiments[1] (Chambless & Ollendick, 2001; Task Force on Promotion and Dissemination of Psychological Procedures, 1995).

The first report of the Division 12 task force, published in 1995, listed 18 empirically supported treatments and was updated several times in subsequent years (e.g., Chambless et al., 1998).[2] The focus, however, was on the adult population, with only a few of these treatments targeting childhood and adolescent disorders. In light of this, the Child Clinical Psychology section of Division 12 organized a new task force aimed at identifying empirically sustained psychological interventions for children and adolescents (Lonigan et al., 1998). Using similar criteria as the first task force, the result of this new task force culminated in a list of 27 empirically supported psychosocial interventions for depression, anxiety disorders, attention

---

[1] For a brief explanation about different research method in psychotherapy, please refer to Leonardi 2017).

[2] Currently, a list of empirically supported treatments, their respective manuals, the clinical research on which they are based, and information on training in these therapies can be found at <www.div12.org/psychological-treatments>. It is worth noting, however, that Division 12 has been replacing the assessment of clinical trials or single-case experiments with systematic review with meta-analysis (Tolin et al., 2015), a method used to synthesize clinical research, explained later.

J. L. Leonardi (✉) · J. L. D. Siqueira
Private Practice, São Paulo, Brazil

© The Author(s), under exclusive license to Springer Nature Switzerland AG 2022
A. S. U. Rossi et al. (eds.), *Clinical Behavior Analysis for Children*, https://doi.org/10.1007/978-3-031-12247-7_6

deficit hyperactivity disorder, oppositional defiant disorder, and autism was published in 1998 in a special issue of the *Journal of Clinical Child Psychology* (which was later renamed the *Journal of Clinical Child and Adolescent Psychology*).

The impact of this work was enormous, which can be seen by the fact that the articles published in this special issue were cited 1140 times in less than 10 years (Silverman & Hinshaw, 2008). In 1999, the Clinical Child Psychology section of Division 12 became its own division – Division 53, currently titled *Society of Clinical Child and Adolescent Psychology* – and since then has been contributing to the development of evidence-based interventions for the prevention and treatment of mental health problems in children and adolescents (Erickson, n.d.).

After a long struggle between various theoretical, conceptual, methodological, and practical perspectives on empirically supported treatments (cf. Leonardi & Meyer, 2015), the American Psychological Association (2006) defined the concept of **evidence-based practice in psychology** as an individualized clinical decision-making process that occurs through the integration of the best available evidence (i.e., therapeutic procedures that are proven to produce positive outcomes and minimize negative outcomes) with clinical expertise (i.e., the ability to formulate the case, apply techniques, monitor progress, establish therapeutic relationship, etc.) in the context of the patient's characteristics, culture, and preferences (i.e., their goals, values, beliefs, context, and clinical status). From this perspective, the three elements of the definition – empirical evidence, professional repertoire, and patient idiosyncrasies – are fundamental in clinical decision-making, so that a professional practice that does not consider the interrelationship between the three components cannot be seen as **evidence-based practice in psychology**.

Waschbusch et al. (2012) point out five characteristics in common in evidence-based interventions for children: (1) they are systematized, extensively studied treatments, described in manuals; (2) they are based on reinforcement programs, both in sessions with therapist and at home and school, to strengthen appropriate behaviors; (3) they involve training of several types of skills, with the main agents of change being parents, teachers, or both; (4) they are behavioral or cognitive behavioral interventions, directed mainly to specific target behaviors; and (5) they typically include procedures to facilitate generalization and maintenance of gains over time.

Implementing evidence-based practice in everyday clinical practice may seem like hard work or even unfeasible, mainly because of the vastness of studies and the heterogeneity among them. In addition, often the therapist has little time available to devote to fundamental questions of critical consumption of research, such as the characteristics of the sample (if it was representative, randomized, and generalizable), the integrity of the procedure (i.e., if the intervention was really executed as planned), the definition of the dependent variable and the way to measure it, the experimental control (if it was adequate and replicable and has clinical meaning), and data analysis (if it assessed intention to treat, if it used appropriate statistical tests, and if it calculated clinical significance), among others. In this sense, it is difficult to know which evidence is reliable and, therefore, which should support the clinical practice, which prevents therapists from reaching a conclusion on the best conduct on each occasion (Norcross et al., 2008).

Many authors (e.g., Schlosser, 2006), taking into account all these difficulties, began to consider the systematic literature review as the first step toward evidence-based practice. This type of study has achieved such relevance because it is a rigorous and replicable protocol that allows comparative analysis of the results of many studies and thus obtains a synthesis of the effects of a certain intervention. Currently, most systematic reviews include meta-analysis, a statistical method that allows mathematically grouping clinical research that used different statistical tests and obtained discrepant results, giving rise to a set of data that represents a summary of the totality of experimental studies (clinical trials or single-case experiments).

Despite the immense prestige it enjoys in evidence-based practice, systematic reviews also present a risk of bias. An example of this is in the process of selecting the research to be included. An article (Kicinski et al., 2015) that examined this type of bias identified that statistically positive results are 27% more likely to be included in review papers in the health area. In addition, the same study found that, in systematic reviews on the safety of drug use, studies that point to a lack of evidence of side effects are 78% more likely to be included in the systematic review than those that reported side effects. To avoid this and other biases, it is essential that the entire data selection and analysis procedure be established and described before the review is conducted. Systematic reviews that respect standardized criteria for the selection and analysis processes of experimental researches may offer essential information about the quality of evidence of a given intervention (Atallah & Castro, 1998). Nevertheless, all this methodological rigor is not necessarily sufficient for the best clinical decision-making.

In 2000, the *Grading of Recommendations, Assessment, Development and Evaluation* (GRADE) working group was created with the purpose of developing a system to assess the quality of evidence and the strength of health recommendations through several factors, such as the methodological quality of the studies, the variability of the results, the balance between desirable and undesirable effects of the intervention, etc. (Guyatt et al., 2011). Currently, GRADE is considered the gold standard in the development of clinical *guidelines*.

Clinical guidelines are recommendations for clinical decision-making that are systematically developed and updated by experts in a given health area, which aim to help professionals offer the best available intervention based on research evidence (Graham et al., 2011). The system proposed by GRADE classifies the quality of evidence into four different levels: high (future research is unlikely to change the confidence in the effect estimates), moderate (future research may have an impact on the estimates), low (future research is very likely to change the estimates), or very low (any effect estimate is very uncertain). Evidence based on randomized clinical trials starts out as high quality, but can be revised if it shows factors such as inconsistencies in results, methodological problems, imprecision, or publication bias (Guyatt et al., 2008).

As for the strength of the recommendations, the GRADE system offers two categories: strong (desirable effects clearly outweigh the undesirable ones or clearly do not) or weak (there is no certainty about the relationship between desirable or undesirable effects). Other factors taken into account when evaluating recommendations are patient preferences and values, as well as estimates of the appropriate use of health system resources, such as cost-effectiveness studies (Guyatt et al., 2008).

The set of clinical guidelines of the UK public health system, the *National Institute for Health and Clinical Excellence* (NICE), is considered one of the most consistent in the world, consisting of more than 120 clinical recommendations based on cost-effectiveness. In 2006, NICE abandoned its traditional classification system to adopt the GRADE system. With this, it began to adopt the practice of assessing confidence in effect estimates for each outcome, weighing both desirable and undesirable outcomes and costs, then generating a judgment on the strength of the recommendation (Thornton et al., 2013).

The NICE guidelines establish recommendations for the most appropriate services for most people with a particular diagnosis, condition, need, or belonging to a particular social group. It also recommends ways to promote and protect health and prevent illness and ways to configure health and social services. Finally, it also establishes how public organizations can improve the quality of health services[3]. With regard to child and adolescent health, NICE currently offers a total of 73 guidelines, covering everything from cochlear implants to fevers in under-5s.

This chapter aims to present a synthesis of the guidelines of NICE and Division 53 – *Society of Clinical Child and Adolescent Psychology* – of the *American Psychological Association* regarding psychological intervention practices in childhood and adolescence. In this sense, the text does not describe the elements and techniques that make up each intervention but offers a kind of guide so that the reader can more easily locate the empirically supported treatments for different clinical pictures.

Depression

The NICE clinical guidelines for depression in children and adolescents adopt a five-step model. The first step establishes that primary care health professionals are trained to identify symptoms of depression and assess risk factors, referring the child to mental health services when necessary. The second step refers to the abilities of health professionals specialized in depression to assess the referred children, using as tools interview instruments such as *Kiddie Schedule for Affective Disorders and Schizophrenia* [K-SADS] or *Child and Adolescent Psychiatric Assessment* [CAPA] and also nonverbal mood assessment in younger children. Of the two tools, only the K-SADS was translated and validated for the Brazilian population (Brasil, 2003).

For children with mild depression (step 3), NICE recommends a "watchful waiting" of 4 weeks after the first assessment. If symptoms have not remitted, nondirective supportive therapy, cognitive behavioral therapy (CBT) group, or guided self-help are offered as options for a limited period between 2 and 3 months.

---

[3] At: <www.nice.org.uk/process/pmg20/chapter/introduction-and-overview>

Children with moderate to severe depression (steps 4 and 5) should be offered specific psychological therapy for at least 3 months. NICE does not indicate a specific psychological approach and proposes that, in the initial period of treatment, it should be explained to the child and family members that there is no superiority relationship between psychological therapies. If the child is unresponsive to treatment after six sessions, referral for multidisciplinary assessment is considered to consider alternative treatment for the child or additional therapy for the parents. In children 5 to 11 years old who are unresponsive to psychotherapy, one may cautiously consider the use of an antidepressant (National Institute for Health and Care Excellence, 2019).

The *American Psychological Association*'s Division 53 differs from NICE in that it places the major psychological approaches for depression in children at different ranks regarding the level of evidence[4]. Group CBT (comprehensive or technology-assisted) and behavioral therapy are classified as *might work*. Individual CBT, psychodynamic therapy, and family intervention are classified as "experimental," that is, one level below on the scale (Weersing et al., 2017).

Despite the high prevalence rate and devastating effects of depression in children, there is little research regarding empirically supported treatments and issues such as comorbidity, family involvement, type of treatment (group vs. individual), and relapse prevention (Cummings & Fristad, 2008). A recent systematic review article (Weersing et al., 2017) concluded that the evidence for depression treatments for children is notably weaker than interventions for adolescents, with no treatment reaching "well-established" status.

There are numerous differences between the studies included in the systematic reviews that support the guidelines. Cummings and Fristad (2008) identified behavioral and cognitive techniques present in most of them. Among the behavioral techniques, exposure, contingency management, scheduling of activities, and relaxation training are highlighted. Among the cognitive techniques, the authors mention self-monitoring, identification of beliefs, and cognitive restructuring. In addition, such interventions seek to help the child in social relationships, offering training in social skills, verbal and nonverbal communication, and problem-solving. Most interventions also work with children's family members.

Attention Deficit Hyperactivity Disorder (ADHD)

The NICE clinical guidelines for treatment of ADHD are divided between children under 5 years and above this age. For children under 5 years, a parent coaching focus group is recommended as a first line of treatment. If symptoms are still having

---

[4] Division 53 classifies the interventions into five categories, according to their respective levels of effectiveness. The categories are (1) works *well*, (2) *works*, (3) *might work*, (4) *experimental*, and (5) *tested and does not work*.

a major impact on the child's life after coaching, consultation with a physician specializing in childhood ADHD is suggested.

For children older than 5 years, the recommendation is to provide information about ADHD as well as additional support for parents, including education and information about the disorder, advice on parenting strategies, and linking to school (with consent). The recommendation is that both parents participate. Medications are only recommended if symptoms are still significantly impacting the child's life even after environmental changes. For children who have benefited from medication but still have significant difficulties, CBT for children with ADHD is considered (National Institute for Health and Care Excellence, 2018).

In the clinical guidelines of the American Psychological Association Division 53, the interventions with the highest level of scientific evidence (level 1: *works well*) are behavioral interventions. Interventions with combined medication training and behavioral therapy are one level below (*works*), and neurofeedback training is classified as level 3 (*might work*) (Evans et al., 2014).

The most frequent empirically supported interventions in ADHD are behavior change strategies through parent training and school-based interventions (Pelham Jr. et al., 2017). Both typically include ADHD psychoeducation for parents and teachers to teach them to identify and praise appropriate behaviors and consistently use appropriate consequences for disruptive behaviors, as well as to help parents and teachers structure the school and home environment and generate realistic expectations (Hoza et al., 2008).

Other empirically supported treatment resources for ADHD are summer programs. Such programs are geared toward children ages 3 to 16 and generally last 7 to 8 weeks, 8 to 9 hours per day. Some of the strategies used are a scoring system for appropriate behavior, social reinforcement in the form of public praise or recognition, daily record cards, "prudent punishment," medical assessment, and school skills training (Pelham Jr. et al., 2017).

Autism

According to NICE guidelines, children with autism and their families should receive detailed information about autism and its treatment from the time of diagnosis, in a manner appropriate to their stage of development. Some interventions are not recommended under any circumstances: neurofeedback, auditory integration training, secretin, chelation therapy, and hyperbaric oxygen therapy.

Regarding problem behaviors, the initial recommendations are to anticipate and prevent them by identifying the factors that increase the likelihood of occurrence, for example, communication difficulties, body conditions (such as gastrointestinal problems and pain) or emotional conditions (anxiety, depression, etc.), noise levels, or lights, among others. The next step is to offer some possible interventions.

If specific aspects that cause the problem behaviors are not identified, a psychosocial intervention based on functional behavior analysis is recommended as the first line of treatment. The interventions should, among other things, clearly identify the target behaviors, focus on quality of life outcomes, and access and modify environmental factors, taking into account the child's developmental stage (National Institute for Health and Care Excellence, 2013a). When psychosocial interventions are not effective, the use of antipsychotics is considered.

In relation to the *American Psychological Association*'s Division 53 classifications of empirically supported treatments, applied behavior analysis (commonly referred to as "ABA") has resources divided into three different levels of evidence. Classified as level 1 (*works well*) are tailoring interventions according to IQ or developmental level and joint engagement in playful activities with caregivers and teachers. Among the interventions indicated as level 2 (*works well*) are the use of figures and symbols to make requests, imitation, language, and cognitive skills, among others. Among the interventions classified as level 3 (*might work*) are training in social skills rated by the teacher and training in the use of spoken words to engage or make requests and engagement with objects in the interaction with teachers and others (Smith & Iadarola, 2015).

It is important to note that, from this perspective, the term ABA refers to a philosophical, theoretical, and technical basis from which different interventions derive, such as DTT (*discrete trial training*), IT (*incidental training*), and PRT (*pivotal response training*). Among the common characteristics are the constant measurement of operationally defined behaviors, the systematic use of reinforcers, the basis in functional analysis, and the emphasis on generalization of learned skills (cf. Cooper et al., 2007).

Obsessive Compulsive Disorder (OCD)

The NICE guidelines for OCD present different recommendations depending on the intensity of symptoms and the degree of impairment experienced. When there is a mild level of impairment, guided self-help for children is recommended, as well as support and information for parents and caregivers. When the impairment caused by the disorder is greater, the recommendation is CBT, including exposure with response prevention, involving family members and caregivers, and adapted to the developmental stage of the child.

According to NICE, treatment should include a good therapeutic alliance, maintain optimism in the child and family, identify key treatment targets, engage the family and caregivers especially in exposure with response prevention (encouraging the return of the technique if new symptoms appear after the end of treatment), and involve teachers and other health professionals (National Institute for Health and Care Excellence, 2005).

Among the psychotherapeutic treatments listed by the *American Psychological Association* Division 53, individual CBT is categorized as level 2 evidence (*works*). Group CBT is one level below that (*might work*). At level 4 (experimental) is technology-based CBT, such as treatment through online social networks (Freeman et al., 2014). The main resources used in CBT for OCD are exposure with response prevention, cognitive techniques, and family involvement.

Thus, it can be concluded that treatment is based on behavioral and cognitive conceptualizations of the disorder, combining exposure and response prevention techniques with cognitive restructuring (Franklin et al., 2017; Storch et al., 2008).

Anxiety

In recent decades, several treatments have been developed specifically for the treatment of anxiety in children. These have varying levels of evidence for efficacy (Silverman & Pina, 2008). However, NICE does not have a more comprehensive category for anxiety in children, although there are guidelines for social anxiety. As general principles for the treatment of this diagnosis, regular clinician supervision, use of outcome measures, engagement in monitoring, assessment of treatment adherence, and clinician competence are recommended. Regarding the approach, NICE recommends CBT focused on social anxiety for children as the most recommended, always considering the active involvement of parents and caregivers in treatment (National Institute for Health and Care Excellence, 2013b).

In the clinical guidelines of Division 53 of the *American Psychological Association*, six interventions were included in level 1, that is, in the category of treatments with the highest level of scientific evidence (level 1: *works well*): CBT, exposure techniques, modeling, CBT with parents, patient psychoeducation, and CBT combined with medication. One level below (*works*) are family psychoeducation, relaxation, assertiveness training, attention control, CBT for parents and children, cultural *storytelling*, hypnosis, and stress inoculation (Higa-McMillan et al., 2016). It is worth noting that most CBT-based treatments for anxiety include psychoeducation, somatic symptom management skills, cognitive restructuring, gradual exposure to feared situations, and relapse prevention plans (Kendall et al., 2017).

Disruptive Disorders

In this category, there are mainly two diagnoses: oppositional defiant disorder (ODD) and conduct disorder. NICE guidelines initially recommend selective prevention, where children at higher risk (low school performance, impulsivity, parental contact with criminal justice, abuse, low education, and low family income) are identified and offered preventive interventions such as emotional learning in the classroom and problem-solving programs.

The second point discussed in the guidelines is evaluation at two levels. The first level takes place in diverse *settings*, such as general health and social care systems, educational settings, and the justice system, among others. The second level is a comprehensive assessment conducted by a mental health or social care professional, which should take into account factors such as patterns of negativity, hostility or challenging behavior, functioning at home and school and with friends, parenting quality, and history of some other mental or physical problem. It should also investigate learning difficulties, disabilities, neurodevelopmental conditions such as autism or ADHD, neurological disorders such as epilepsy or motor impairment, substance abuse, or communication disorders. The assessment should also make use of instruments and include an interview with parents/carers.

As for interventions for ODD or conduct disorder, the main NICE recommendation is parent training programs. The groups should have 10 to 12 parents and are composed of 10 to 16 sessions of 90 to 120 minutes duration. Interventions are based on social learning, using modeling, behavioral rehearsal, and feedback to improve parenting skills. Ideally, both parents should be involved in the program (National Institute for Health and Care Excellence, 2017).

In the *American Psychological Association*'s Division 53 evaluation of empirically supported treatments, the interventions with the highest level of evidence (*works well*) are the combined treatments of behavioral therapy, CBT, and family therapy, such as multisystemic therapy or *Treatment Foster Care Oregon* (TFCO). Treatments that involve CBT or behavioral therapy alone or even skills training all have lower levels of evidence of effectiveness (Kaminski & Claussen, 2017).

Final Considerations

This chapter has presented a synthesis of the research evidence-based recommendations offered by NICE and the *American Psychological Association*'s Division 53 on the best psychological treatments for some clinical conditions in children and adolescents. It is up to the reader interested in implementing these interventions to appropriate each of them in their respective manuals (books that describe step by step how to perform them). In addition, we suggest reading compendia that deepen the topics covered in this chapter and describe empirically supported interventions for other problems (posttraumatic stress, enuresis and encopresis, eating disorders, self-mutilation, chemical dependence, suicide, etc.). Some examples are the following books:

- Weisz, J. R., & Kazdin, A. E. (Orgs.). (2017). *Evidenced-based psychotherapies for children and adolescents*. Guilford.
- Theodore, L. A. (Org.). (2016). *Handbook of evidence-based interventions for children and adolescents*. Springer.
- Sturmey, P., & Hersen, M. (Orgs.). (2012). *Handbook of evidence-based practice in clinical psychology: Child and adolescent disorders*. Hoboken: Wiley.

In summary, it is hoped that this chapter has impelled the reader to act according to the model of evidence-based practice in psychology in the prevention and treatment of mental health problems in children and adolescents.

References

American Psychological Association. (2006). Evidence-based practice in psychology: APA presidential task force on evidence-based practice. *American Psychologist, 61*, 271–285.

Atallah, A. N., & Castro, A. A. (1998). Revisão sistemática da literatura e metanálise: a melhor forma de evidência para tomada de decisão em saúde e a maneira mais rápida de atualização terapêutica. Em A. N. Atallah & A. A. Castro (Orgs.), *Evidências para melhores decisões clínicas* (pp. 20–28). Lemos Editorial.

Brasil, H. H. A. (2003). *Desenvolvimento da versão brasileira da K-SADS-PL* (Schudule for affective disorders and schizophrenia for school aged children present and lifetime version) e estudo de suas propriedades psicométricas. 301 f. (v. 1 e 2) p. Tese (Doutorado em Ciências) – Escola Paulista de Medicina, Universidade Federal de São Paulo, 2003.

Chambless, D. L. (1993). *Task force on promotion and dissemination of psychological procedures: A report adopted by the Division 12 Board.* American Psychological Association. http://www.apa.org/divisions/div12/est/chamble2.pdf

Chambless, D., & Ollendick, T. (2001). Empirically supported psychological interventions: Controversies and evidence. *Annual Review of Psychology, 52*, 685–716.

Chambless, D. L., Baker, M., Baucom, D. H., Beutler, L. E., Calhoun, K. S., Crits-Christoph, P., & Woody, S. R. (1998). Update on empirically validated therapies, II. *The Clinical Psychologist, 51*, 3–16.

Cooper, J. O., Heron, T. E., & Heward, W. L. (2007). *Applied Behavior Analysis* (2nd ed.). Pearson Prentice Hall.

Cummings, C. M., & Fristad, M. A. (2008). Mood disorders in childhood. Em R. G. Steele, D. T. Elkin & M. Roberts (Orgs.), *Handbook of evidence-based therapies for children and adolescents: Bridging science and practice* (pp. 145–160). Springer.

Erickson, M. (n.d.). *A brief history of the Society of Clinical Child and Adolescent Psychology (SCCAP) from Section 1, APA Division 12, status through APA Division 53 status.* Retirado de http://sccap53.org/about-us/history/history-of-division-53

Evans, S. W., Owens, J. S., & Bunford, N. (2014). Evidence-based psychosocial treatments for children and adolescents with attention-deficit/hyperactivity disorder. *Journal of Clinical Child & Adolescent Psychology, 43*, 527–551.

Franklin, M. E., Morris, S. H., Freeman, J. B., & March, J. S. (2017). Treating pediatric obsessive-compulsive disorder in children: Using exposure-based cognitive-behavioral therapy. Em J. R. Weisz & A. E. Kazdin (Orgs.), *Evidenced-based psychotherapies for children and adolescents* (pp. 35–48). Guilford.

Freeman, J., Garcia, A., Frank, H., Benito, K., Conelea, C., Walther, M., & Edmunds, J. (2014). Evidence base update for psychosocial treatments for pediatric obsessive-compulsive disorder. *Journal of Clinical Child & Adolescent Psychology, 43*, 7–26.

Graham, R., Mancher, M., Wolman, D. M., Greenfield, S., & Steinberg, E. (Orgs.). (2011). *Clinical practice guidelines we can trust.* Institute of Medicine, National Academies Press.

Guyatt, G. H., Oxman, A. D., Vist, G. E., Kunz, R., Falck-Ytter, Y., Alonso-Coello, P., & Schünemann, H. J. (2008). GRADE: An emerging consensus on rating quality of evidence and strength of recommendations. *BMJ, 336*, 924–926.

Guyatt, G. H., Oxman, A. D., Schünemann, H. J., Tugwell, P., & Knottnerus, A. (2011). GRADE guidelines: A new series of articles in the *Journal of Clinical Epidemiology*. *Journal of Clinical Epidemiology, 64*, 380–382.

Higa-McMillan, C. K., Francis, S. E., Rith-Najarian, L., & Chorpita, B. F. (2016). Evidence base update: 50 years of research on treatment for child and adolescent anxiety. *Journal of Clinical Child & Adolescent Psychology, 45*, 91–113.

Hoza, B., Kaiser, N., & Hurt, E. (2008). Evidence-based treatments for attention-deficit/hyperactivity disorder (ADHD). Em R. G. Steele, D. T. Elkin, & M. Roberts (Orgs.), *Handbook of evidence-based therapies for children and adolescents: Bridging science and practice* (pp. 197–220). Springer.

Kaminski, J. W., & Claussen, A. H. (2017). Evidence base update for psychosocial treatments for disruptive behaviors in children. *Journal of Clinical Child & Adolescent Psychology, 46,* 477–499.

Kendall, P. C., Crawford, E. A., Kagan, E. R., Furr, J. M., & Podell, J. L. (2017). Child-focused treatment for anxiety. Em J. R. Weisz & A. E. Kazdin (Orgs.), *Evidenced-based psychotherapies for children and adolescents* (pp. 17–34). Guilford.

Kicinski, M., Springate, D. A., & Kontopantelis, E. (2015). Publication bias in meta-analyses from the Cochrane database of systematic reviews. *Statistics in Medicine, 34,* 2781–2793.

Leonardi, J. L. (2017). Métodos de pesquisa para o estabelecimento da eficácia das psicoterapias. *Interação em Psicologia, 21,* 176–186.

Leonardi, J. L., & Meyer, S. B. (2015). Prática baseada em evidências em psicologia e a história da busca pelas provas empíricas da eficácia das psicoterapias. *Psicologia: Ciência e Profissão, 35,* 1139–1156.

Lonigan, C., Elbert, J. C., & Johnson, S. B. (1998). Empirically supported psychosocial interventions for children: An overview. *Journal of Clinical Child Psychology, 27,* 138–145.

National Institute for Health and Care Excellence. (2005). *Obsessive-compulsive disorder and body dysmorphic disorder: Treatment* (NICE guideline No. 31). http://www.nice.org.uk/guidance/cg31

National Institute for Health and Care Excellence. (2013a). *Autism spectrum disorder in under 19s: Support and management* (NICE guideline No. 170). https://www.nice.org.uk/guidance/cg170

National Institute for Health and Care Excellence. (2013b). *Social anxiety disorder: Recognition, assessment and treatment* (NICE guideline No. 159). http://www.nice.org.uk/guidance/cg159

National Institute for Health and Care Excellence. (2017). *Antisocial behaviour and conduct disorders in children and young people: Recognition and management* (NICE guideline No. 158). https://www.nice.org.uk/guidance/cg158

National Institute for Health and Care Excellence. (2018). *Attention deficit hyperactivity disorder: Diagnosis and management* (NICE guideline No. 87). http://www.nice.org.uk/guidance/NG87

National Institute for Health and Care Excellence. (2019). *Depression in children and young people: Identification and management* (NICE guideline No. 134). http://www.nice.org.uk/guidance/ng134

Norcross, J. C., Hogan, T. P., & Koocher, G. P. (2008). *Clinician's guide to evidence-based practices: Mental health and the addictions.* Oxford University Press.

Pelham, W. E., Jr., Gnagy, E. M., Greiner, A. R., Fabiano, G. A., Waschbusch, D. A., & Koles, E. K. (2017). Summer treatment programs for attention-deficit/hyperactivity disorder. Em J. R. Weisz & A. E. Kazdin (Orgs.), *Evidenced-based psychotherapies for children and adolescents* (pp. 215–234). Guilford.

Schlosser, R. W. (2006). The role of systematic reviews in evidence-based practice, research, and development. *Focus, 15,* 1–4.

Silverman, W. K., & Hinshaw, S. P. (2008). The second special issue on evidence-based psychosocial treatments for children and adolescents: A 10-year update. *Journal of Clinical Child and Adolescent Psychology, 37,* 1–7.

Silverman, W. K., & Pina, A. A. (2008). Psychosocial treatments for phobic and anxiety disorders in youth. Em R. G. Steele, D. T. Elkin, & M. Roberts (Orgs.), *Handbook of evidence-based therapies for children and adolescents: Bridging science and practice* (pp. 65–82). Springer.

Smith, T., & Iadarola, S. (2015). Evidence base update for autism spectrum disorder. *Journal of Clinical Child & Adolescent Psychology, 44,* 897–922.

Storch, E. A., Larson, M., Adkins, J., Geffken, G. R., Murphy, T. K., & Goodman, W. K. (2008). Evidence-based treatment of pediatric obsessive-compulsive disorder. Em R. G. Steele, D. T. Elkin, & M. Roberts (Orgs.), *Handbook of evidence-based therapies for children and adolescents: Bridging science and practice* (pp. 103–120). Springer.

Task Force on Promotion and Dissemination of Psychological Procedures. (1995). Training in and dissemination of empirically-validated psychological treatments: Report and recommendations. *The Clinical Psychologist, 48,* 3–23.

Thornton, J., Alderson, P., Tan, T., Turner, C., Latchem, S., Shaw, E., & Neilson, J. (2013). Introducing GRADE across the NICE clinical guideline program. *Journal of Clinical Epidemiology, 66*, 124–131.

Tolin, D. F., McKay, D., Forman, E. M., Klonsky, E. D., & Thombs, B. D. (2015). Empirically supported treatment: Recommendations for a new model. *Clinical Psychology: Science and Practice, 22*, 317–338.

Waschbusch, D. A., Fabiano, G. A., & Pelham, W. E. (2012). Evidence-based practice in child and adolescent disorders. Em P. Sturmey & M. Hersen (Orgs.), *Handbook of evidence-based practice in clinical psychology: Child and adolescent disorders* (pp. 27–49). Wiley.

Weersing, V. R., Jeffreys, M., Do, M. C. T., Schwartz, K. T., & Bolano, C. (2017). Evidence base update of psychosocial treatments for child and adolescent depression. *Journal of Clinical Child & Adolescent Psychology, 46*, 11–43.

Chapter 7
Functional Play: Ways to Conduct and the Development of Skills of the Clinical Behavior Analyst for Children

Ana Beatriz Chamati and Liane Dahás

Introduction

The beginning of the work of the child behavioral psychologist raises many questions. A considerable part of psychology courses do not teach relevant guidelines for the treatment of children. One of the main differences between adult and child psychotherapy is the constant search for alternative procedures to verbal reporting to access the child's world and for information about the variables that control their behavior.

One of the prerequisites of child care is the use of play as a clinical care tool, a practice also known as play therapy. Thus, psychologists who start attending children end up identifying the importance of play, as well as its effectiveness in the psychotherapy session as one of the most explored tools in psychotherapeutic context to evoke clinically relevant behaviors (CRB1) as described by Kohlenberg and Tsai (1991). In addition, it also plays a key role in clinical intervention and management, which makes it worthy of careful analysis.

According to Rule (2000), child psychotherapy is unique because (1) the child may have difficulty talking about his or her own feelings when they are unpleasant, since his or her behavior has likely been punished, (2) the child may have been poorly taught to name his or her covert behaviors, since the verbal community itself has difficulty establishing this training, (3) the child may fear being disapproved of by the therapist when reporting certain feelings, and (4) the child may fear that what he or she says to the therapist will be reported to his or her parents.

A methodology that has been shown to be effective for children to produce reports is the use of fantasy, games, and drawings. In this way, data collection in child therapy differs greatly from that of therapy with adults, since not only

---

A. B. Chamati · L. Dahás (✉)
Paradigma, Center for Behavioral Sciences and Technology, São Paulo, Brazil

© The Author(s), under exclusive license to Springer Nature Switzerland AG 2022
A. S. U. Rossi et al. (eds.), *Clinical Behavior Analysis for Children*,
https://doi.org/10.1007/978-3-031-12247-7_7

drawings and games are indispensable but also reports from adults with whom the child interacts, such as parents and teachers.

According to Moura and Venturelli (2004), the use of play is also effective for the therapy and the therapist to be paired with enjoyable activities, as well as for the therapist to plan situations in which the client explains antecedents and consequences of observed behaviors. Furthermore, the use of play can be useful to therapist and child analyze together the feasibility of more adaptive behaviors, which could even give the opportunity to practice them within the session.

For gestalt psychotherapist Violet Oaklander, "How she plays tells a lot about how she is in her life" (1978, p. 160). In her book, the author describes various techniques she has used in child care, including play, drawings, storytelling, etc. The psychotherapist can, in fact, use these techniques as a way of collecting data about his client, as well as teaching and training him (behavioral rehearsal) to have more appropriate behaviors in the environment, through activities such as fantasizing that he is another person, drawing, or playing in general.

Concept of Play

If, on the one hand, this chapter presents the possibility of using play with a therapeutic purpose, the most commonly used concept in the Portuguese language for playing means precisely doing something without any practical purpose. According to the definition of Dicionário Aurélio (2018), to play is "(...) [d]ivertise. To amuse oneself with something childish. To joke; to jest. To agitate in a mechanical way. To proceed lightly. To agitate (it is said of the waves)."

We then understood that, in a certain way, using play for psychotherapeutic purposes would make it lose its most central characteristic, that of being the result of spontaneity and lack of teleological biases. This theoretical discussion loses its importance, however, when we rely on a basic premise of radical behaviorism, which is that all behavior has function, even if the person behaving does not know how to describe it (or is not aware of it). Thus, if all behavior has function and if playing is something done spontaneously, we understand the phrase "children do not play at playing, they play for real" (Quintana, 2005, p. 805).

When a child plays house freely, it does not say that she does it to learn how to behave when she is older, in her profession, or when caring for her children; however, it is known that this turns out to be an important function of "imitating adult play" (Papalia et al., 2009, p. 292). Similarly, when children play freely representing the daily activities of their own routine, they tend to reproduce what they live in everyday life. Thus, this chapter presents, explains, and defends functional play, which would be nothing more than to maintain, in psychotherapeutic context, the typical spontaneity of play that occurs outside the office, provided that the psychologist knows how to conduct and describe for himself the functions that the actions of the players are presenting and how to use them for psychotherapy purposes.

Play in Child Development

Play is believed to be a way to develop skills, or in other words, to build knowledge. In several mammalian species, play during the first years of life has survival value. The game of hide-and-seek is common in several cultures around the world (Fernald & O'Neill, 1993), for example. The adult draws the child's attention with exaggerated gestures or sounds, hides behind a cloth or hands, and then reappears emitting specific, usually high-pitched, sounds. In the first 6 months, play primarily involves the adult's attempt to draw the child's attention to the start of play, which becomes less necessary as the months pass; until by age two, the infant is able to initiate play by covering himself or herself or by covering a doll (Rome-Flanders et al., 1995).

Papalia et al. (2009) describe the changes in the hide-and-seek play over the months involving more and more anticipatory responses of the infant to what is expected from the adult, indicating that the experience taught that child to react to what we call expectation. It is also possible that this play teaches him/her skills such as alternating turns during verbal episodes, responding attentively to the action of others, regulating emotions when facing the disappearance of the adult, or even developing the ability to deal with the permanence of objects, as pointed out by the Piagetian theory.

In addition to establishing a bond, play such as "Follow the leader" allows children to learn to coordinate their actions with those of other children, a behavior that enables the development of even more complex games such as "Police and robbers" and "Pike and hide," common in the preschool years (Eckerman & Didow, 1996). Make-believe play allows children to explore different social roles, identify other children's perspectives, and sometimes get in touch with emotions considered uncomfortable.

Culture strongly influences the content and partners of play: in Eastern cultures, for example, make-believe tends to be more cooperative and frequent with caregivers, who use this moment to teach behaviors perceived as appropriate (such as cooperation), while Western children tend to do imaginative play among their peers, developing autonomy and sometimes creating conflict situations, placing less emphasis on group harmony than Eastern children (Farver et al., 1995; Haight et al., 1999).

Gender typification is also, in part, a consequence of childhood play, in which boys and girls learn how their culture expects them to behave: mothers encourage their daughters to talk to them more than their sons (stimulating socialization and the expression of feelings), while fathers play more roughly with their sons than with their daughters (stimulating competition and aggression) (Leaper et al., 1998; Leaper & Smith, 2004). Gender specificities in peer play are also common across cultures and, from an evolutionary perspective, seem to promote training for later developmental periods in which appropriate behaviors for reproduction and survival of that gender should be emitted (Papalia et al., 2009).

As the examples above illustrate, for developmental psychology, children's play leads to the acquisition of skills, from the most basic, such as sensorimotor skills

(Papalia et al., 2009), to more complex ones, which involve verbal behavior, such as predicting the future, describing past events, mathematical concepts, planning, self-control, and cooperative responses. Although permeated with mentalistic explanations, the consumption of this literature allows behavior analysts to understand the importance of play and, therefore, to assume it as a psychotherapeutic practice.

Functional Play

The use of games and toys in clinical behavior analysis for children is relatively recent. The relationship between the child and the toy in psychotherapy has evolved since the child behavior modification (Krumboltz & Krumboltz, 1977), when the child was not considered part of the psychotherapy process and only the parents' complaint was treated without direct and frequent contact with the child (Gadelha & de Menezes, 2004). The behavioral assessment materials were inventories that assessed behaviors and symptoms present in anxiety, depression, aggressiveness, and shyness (Watson & Gresham, 1998). The therapist worked with parents to identify the child's problem behaviors, and their private events were not part of the complaint analysis (Conte & Regra, 2000). Experimental practices from laboratories were also used to modify the child's problem behaviors (Conte & Regra, 2000). Since the psychologist had no contact with the child, it was not possible to assess whether the parents' verbal report about their children corresponded with what the child presented in clinical context. Thus, play was far from being a tool for behavioral assessment and intervention, since the child was not even part of the psychotherapeutic process.

In 1960, child behavior therapy became a psychotherapeutic model (Gadelha & de Menezes, 2004). The child became the protagonist in the psychotherapeutic process, and his behavior began to be analyzed functionally in relation to his environment, such as parents, school, and peers (Gadelha & de Menezes, 2004). With these changes in the configuration of child therapy, the psychologist began to have direct contact with the child, and this relationship then became the target of functional analysis (Conte & Regra, 2000).

Thus, the need arose to accurately describe the behavior of the child psychologist, who identifies antecedents, responses, and consequences that make up a class of responses through what we call play. He also identifies variables that guide decision-making about the path to be followed. It is through play that the therapist evaluates the child's behavior and intervenes to modify what is presented as a complaint.

Although the definition of play is not precise within behavior analysis, it cannot be neglected that children play (De Rose & Gil, 2003). Playing requires spontaneity and pleasure and, whether done in a planned or free manner, is part of child development, presenting itself as one of the child's ways of communicating. In play, the child expresses feelings, wishes, and desires that often are not expressed verbally (De Rose & Gil, 2003).

Exploring the possibility of understanding what play behavior is, we cannot consider only the topography of the response. To this end, behavior analysts take into account the notion of reinforcing contingencies, which allows exploring the function of playing in child development (De Rose & Gil, 2003). Our behaviors are selected by the consequences produced in the environment (Skinner, 1953). Children need to learn to play, and, to do so, a wide variety of operant behaviors are necessary (De Rose & Gil, 2003). A baby lying in the crib, when swinging his arm, hits the hanging mobile and produces the sound of a song. This sound is a reinforcing consequence for the baby's behavior, so the probability that he will again swing his arm to produce the noise may increase. We then say that the baby is playing in his crib. We call this whole contingency play.

Toys can be discriminative stimuli, models, instructions, and consequences, and with them, from the child's initial repertoire, it is possible to refine behaviors and learn new ones. Thus, we use play and toys as an evaluation and intervention method, since it is possible to evaluate problem behavior and install new behaviors, modifying the child's relationship with the environment. Therefore, once the child has acquired a minimum repertoire to participate in play, it opens wide perspectives to refine and diversify the individual's repertoire in its motor, cognitive, affective, social, and verbal aspects (De Rose & Gil, 2003).

It's common to see children spontaneously playing with something that we don't necessarily call a toy. A class of stimuli can be called a toy if, in the presence of these stimuli, the child emits a single play response. When, in front of an object, the child manipulates, touches, handles, explores, stacks, looks, and puts in the mouth, among other actions, that's when we say she is playing. Thus, a toy is an instrument of the learning process, and playing is also a possibility to learn new behaviors in the face of certain stimuli. When recording the observation of playing behavior, we should pay attention to the most accurate behavioral description possible. It is worth remembering that in trying to propose a format for using play as a working tool in child therapy, we must never forget the individual analysis of each peculiar situation involving play, because two children may present the same topography in a given play, having different functions in each case.

When playing, free from any punitive audience, the child presents a behavioral repertoire related to his life story and expresses his feelings, values, secrets, and intimacy. Playing is a class of responses subject to functional analysis and behavioral management just like any other class of responses. Through play, children develop their ability to observe and describe what happens around them, increasing their knowledge of themselves and of others. When she plays, she shows her world and the behaviors she learned to relate to others. When she plays, the child is herself.

In general, playing freely, without demand, may be easy for some. On the other hand, functional play as a resource for the behavior analyst is a more complex skill that requires learning, training, study, supervision with more experienced therapists, and exposure to the universe of children, among others. All this brings more security in clinical performance for the use of any playful tool, forming an important baggage over the years of work.

Thus, we understand that functional play in the assessment phase involves the emission of responses typical of the behavioral repertoire of the child under analysis, allowing clinical behavior analysis for children to analyze the functions of such responses, and can also be used as an aid in the installation of new repertoire during the intervention phase[1]. Let's list some functions of play for the psychotherapist: (1) to bond with the child so that he/she will want to return for future sessions; (2) bring up themes possibly paired with aversive situations and that, therefore, elicit feelings such as anger, sadness, anguish, jealousy, etc.; (3) access the child's relationship with his environment, whether private or public; (4) evaluate the complaint; (5) install a new response; and (6) teach the child to observe antecedents and consequents of his responses, to help him identify the occurrence of similar behaviors in the natural environment.

Play as a Method of Assessment and Intervention

It is common for beginning therapists to report the feeling that they are just playing, without a clear objective, and that they are not using the tool of play as a method of assessment and intervention. Therefore, one must always keep in mind the following question: why and for what purpose am I doing this now? Whenever we use functional analysis structuring sessions, in an attempt to manage the target behavior, we are directing the play with psychotherapeutic function. We should always use play as part of this logic.

We will highlight two objectives presented above: playing as an assessment method and playing as an intervention method. At the beginning of the therapeutic process with the child, after the initial interview with the parents, the behavioral assessment phase begins. It is suggested that the first sessions be almost entirely intervention-free on the part of the psychotherapist. Obviously, if a child is about to hurt himself, take a risk, or break some material in the room, one should assess how safe and necessary it is to leave the child free to explore the environment. The behavioral assessment phase is most intense in the first four or five sessions, but is present throughout the psychotherapy process, since we are always evaluating the effect of interventions and clinical management strategies, as well as the maintenance of new behaviors.

In the first sessions, we should expose the child to different materials and situations. The focus is on observing how the child relates to the treatment room and therapist, rather than manipulating variables. What are the correspondences between the behavioral repertoire presented by the child and what the parents described? What is different from what the parents described? It is necessary that the therapist has knowledge of child development to evaluate any and all behaviors that the child

---

[1] It is possible that understanding the concept of a higher order (or second order) class of behavior may help the clinical behavior analysis for children in training to generalize their functional play repertoire. For further exploration, we suggest reading the ninth chapter of Catania (1999).

presents and that together may indicate some alteration in the development typically observed.

Some examples of behaviors to be evaluated are eye contact with the interlocutor; greeting when arriving for the session, verbally or with hug or kiss on the cheek gestures; literality; rigidity/flexibility; ability to play individually and with others, competing or cooperating; way of organizing the room, the game, and objects; drawings; appropriation of the therapeutic space; way of sitting; verbalizations about the room; preferences for activities and games; and if he tries new games. Everything the child does should be evaluated, and everything in the room can be a discriminative stimulus that evokes and/or elicits responses relevant to the clinical context.

After the evaluation phase, the intervention phase begins. This phase is planned to structure games that allow the child to learn alternative responses to the problem behavior presented, such as hitting, swearing, yelling, crying, difficulty expressing what they are feeling, and breaking rules, among others. When playing, the child exhibits the problem behavior and, through the therapist's intervention and management, learns alternative responses more adapted to the social context. The therapist should teach the child to understand that the problem is not feeling the emotions that the context elicits but how he/she experiences and expresses these emotions in the world. Thus, learning alternative ways of expressing emotions is a key goal of the psychotherapy process.

Listed below are some variables that should be taken into consideration by the therapist when choosing the play activity to be used:

(1) Target behavior selected for intervention and (2) its possible controlling variables (identification of antecedent and consequent that control the child's behavior): the initial sessions with the parents already bring numerous hypotheses about variables that maintain the complaint to be checked in the sessions with the child. Listing these responses is the first step to thinking of games capable of evoking them. It is also important to vary the play contexts to verify in which the problem behavior is more frequent. Children who arrive with a previous psychiatric diagnosis or if it is possible to identify in the symptoms described by their parents the possibility of a psychiatric diagnosis already bring the hints about the behaviors to focus on in child therapy. For example, children diagnosed with attention deficit hyperactivity disorder (ADHD) or oppositional defiant disorder (ODD) need to have their self-control and rule-following repertoires evaluated.

In this sense, any game with rules can be very effective in establishing both natural, winning the game, and arbitrary, therapist praise for having obeyed pre-established rules, consequences of behavior. Another function of a game may be to bring the child closer to an aversive theme, for example, using a game that contains the picture of a dog to evoke behaviors of a child who the parents described as someone who is afraid of dogs.

Baking a cake at home or making Jell-O can be medium-term consequence teaching contingencies, teaching the child to wait (the consequence of trying to eat them ahead of time tends to be aversive). Another possibility is to guide parents to make allowance available, educating children to think with spending categories such as short, medium, and long term, associating them with the child's reality spending and desires. To do so, three boxes can be built (in session or at home with the parents) to help separate spending criteria, establishing the notion of monetary values, magnitudes of reinforcing value, and importance for the delay of the consequence. In session, it is possible to have a surprise box whose contents are only revealed at the end of the session.

(3) Activity appropriate to what is previously known about the child's repertoire and developmental stage: when presenting any activity to the child, it is important to know previously if it is appropriate for his/her age. A 12-year-old child will hardly wish to play with dolls and a house in session. In the same way, a 4-year-old child will hardly sit on the couch in the treatment room and discuss with linear speech and relevant details about possible complaints for treatment during the therapeutic process. It is necessary to take into consideration what the literature describes about what is appropriate for each age.

(4) Preferences and tastes of each child: the therapist should seek to know the children's universe for each age group: characters, sticker albums, movies, toys, etc. When not aware of something brought by the client, it is expected that the clinical behavior analyst for children will show interest, seeking to understand during the session or, even outside it, the context in which the toy/personage appears in the child's imaginary, and thus be able to use it for analysis or even intervention purposes.

(5) Degree of aversiveness of the activity: it is common that some activities, although unpleasant or unwanted by the child, are important for intervention, such as the presentation of a new game or a book with longer texts. In these cases, it is suggested to establish the *fade-in* procedure of the activity, i.e., that it be suggested and inserted gradually, allowing habituation of unpleasant responders and pairing the activity with some motivational stimulation (characters, costumes, songs).

The Premack principle (Catania, 1999) can also be used: it consists of presenting to the patient the possibility of engaging in an aversive activity with the possibility of engaging in another highly reinforcing activity. One can propose a hunt for pictures previously hidden in the office, a subsequent session involving a high-magnitude reinforcer, such as one outside the office to meet the therapist's pet, or even arrange for the child to borrow a toy from the office, which generates the teaching of trust, responsibility, and care, among others.

(6) Division of session time between the moment when the therapist proposes an activity and the moment when the client can propose what will be done: this is usually done in order to establish a routine for the therapeutic environment, usually beginning with an activity proposed by the therapist with a specific objective (which may be orally explained to the child, depending on the function) and ending with something chosen by the client. It is important to remember that the need for this division (or even this order) should be related to the management/intervention in each case. In some cases, it will be necessary to develop autonomy and decision-making in some children and especially in adolescents. In this case, it would be more advisable to allow them to have a more active participation in the choice of activities. In cases where the child shows natural motivation for the activities

presented by the therapist, as well as talking about the complaints related to the problem behavior, this division is not necessary.

(7) Availability of resources (material, time, space): there are several possibilities of materials for the development of play. We can use games, dolls, and play dough, create activities applied to therapeutic objectives, adapt the material according to the client's demand, and change the rules of games for specific purposes modifying the initial proposal, such as repeated album pictures used as a memory game.

(8) Unforeseen events during the session: one of the greatest difficulties of therapists, especially the less experienced, is to deal with unforeseen events during the session. Understanding that functional analysis guides our interventions and guides our decisions may assure the beginning therapist the possibility of experimenting with creating a playful situation adequate to the new context, maintaining the initial objective of the session or even changing it to another that emerges. All this is sometimes done in the company of the child itself. If the planning to read a book that will explore social skills repertoire does not make sense because the child came to the clinic crying after learning that the dog is sick, for example, the therapist should be sensitive to the demand brought, accept the suffering, and redirect the course of the session (e.g., to tasks of expressing emotions, and problem-solving). Many times, the therapist plays with the attachment function, and, if this is clear in the functional analysis, the therapist, beginner or experienced, will feel safe.

Below are some play resources for the child therapist and their clinical management possibilities:

(a) Board and card games: allow teaching obedience to pre-established rules, modifying rules to adapt to the needs of the case, evaluating the ability to cooperate, and using parts of the game with another function, for example, making the pins into interacting characters. We should be careful with games that teach theoretically about social and socioemotional skills, because children may not be interested. We also run the risk of the child verbalizing correctly what empathy or cooperation is, but the verbal discourse does not correspond with the child's doing/living outside the clinic.

(b) Fantasy: it is one of the richest resources with infants and toddlers. An imaginary friend allows bringing direction to some problem behavior in session, explores the capacity of creativity and problem-solving, and stimulates the development of social repertoire. The "fairy door"[2], which can be made by the therapist and introduced into the treatment room, functions as a possibility to train social repertoire and to talk about feelings and problems to the therapist in an indirect manner, as the child can write and draw for the fairy. Waiting for the fairy's response, which may occur in the following week's session or 2 or

---

[2] The fairy door is a small wooden door (or other material, like EVA, for example) that is used by the first author to connect the real world with an imaginary world of the child, bringing several possibilities of intervention. The child can write to the fairy about something they have difficulty with, which may or may not be part of the complaint, and they can share with the fairy some situation they have experienced. The child's drawing or letter is answered by the fairy when she passes by to pick up what the children leave for her, without having a certain day or time.

3 weeks later, also allows the child to develop his/her self-control and waiting repertoire.

Cloth dolls also stimulate fantasy: through interaction between the characters, we teach children to make functional analysis of the behavior of the characters and of themselves, and we can represent roles of difficult situations for the child assessing and creating new social repertoire. Playing with dolls involves exploring the natural environment in a non-aversive way and also emotional expression, representing the child's real environment, such as two houses in the case of separated parents. Many children speak through the dolls what they cannot speak directly to the therapist. It is possible for both the therapist to visualize the way the child manipulates the dolls in order to reproduce the home environment and for the therapist to represent situations from the child's life that he/she has knowledge of in order to analyze how the child reacts. The therapist can stimulate the child's critical thinking by asking what he thinks about the way the doll acted or how he is feeling.

The activity of playing at being the "problem detective," another possibility using the resource of fantasy, stimulates problem-solving step by step and also creativity, because the child asks himself questions, as if he were a detective, and, with each answer, creates a new question in an attempt to reach the final objective. It is noteworthy that it is even possible to have a magnifying glass in the office and interpret with the child as a detective.

(c) Children's books: these are rich tools and allow countless possibilities, such as observing the child's reading of both words and images, presenting an important theme for the psychotherapeutic process, exploring the attitude of the characters, and reflecting if the child knows someone who resembles a character in the book, among others.
(d) Play dough: allows exploring basic motor skills, fantasy with the construction or creation of objects, characters, food, identification, and naming of feelings in front of the material represented by the dough.
(e) Activities with paper, crayons, and markers: the possibilities are endless. It is possible to make free drawings, family drawings, and family drawings representing an animal for each family member or a goal, based on the individual characteristics of each family member; create stories from the drawings; and build comics with the children, decreasing or increasing the response cost of the child involving the participation of the therapist.

Conclusion

The clinical behavior analyst for children in training often enters this playful universe in such a pleasurable, genuine, and spontaneous way that we sometimes hear from students who feel in doubt whether they are playing to work or working to play. At this moment, our achievement of having contributed to the training of a child therapist becomes clear, leaving us with the hope that he/she will remain in constant search for learning and improvement of his/her abilities to play functionally.

This chapter aimed to present the countless possibilities of creativity of management and clinical intervention in the clinical behavior analysis for children. Suggestions and ideas were presented, without exhausting by any means the infinite range of creative possibilities within the universe of functional play. It is important for the psychotherapist, based on his studies, supervision, reading, and clinical experience, among others, to create his own way of working, always considering that if there is a behavioral function, within ethical limits, we can act.

References

Catania, A. C. (1999). *Aprendizagem: Comportamento, linguagem e cognição* (D. G. Souza, trad. coord.). Artes Médicas.
Conte, F. C. S., & Regra, J. A. G. (2000). A psicoterapia comportamental infantil: novos aspectos. In E. F. M. Silvares (Ed.), *Estudos de caso em psicologia clínica comportamental infantil* (pp. 79–13). Papirus.
De Rose, J. C. C., & Gil, M. S. C. A. (2003). Para uma análise do brincar e sua função educacional. In M. Z. Brandão (Ed.), *Sobre comportamento e cognição: a história e os avanços, a seleção por consequências em ação* (Vol. 11, pp. 373–382). ESETed.
Dicionário Aurélio Online. (2018). https://dicionariodoaurelio.com/brincar
Eckerman, C. O., & Didow, S. M. (1996). Nonverbal imitation and toddlers' mastery of verbal means of achieving coordinated action. *Developmental Psychology, 32*, 141–152.
Farver, J. A. M., Kim, Y. K., & Lee, Y. (1995). Cultural differences in Korean and Anglo-American preschoolers' social interaction and play behavior. *Child Development, 66*, 1088–1099.
Fernald, A., & O'Neill, D. K. (1993). Peekaboo across cultures: How mothers and infants play with voices, faces, and expectations. In K. MacDonald (Ed.), *Parent-child play*. State University of New York Press.
Gadelha, Y. A., & de Menezes, I. N. (2004). Estratégias lúdicas na relação terapêutica com crianças na terapia comportamental. *Universitas: Ciências da saúde, 2*(1), 57–68.
Haight, W. L., Wang, X. L., Fung, H. H., Williams, K., & Mintz, J. (1999). Universal, developmental, and variable aspects of young children's play: A cross-cultural comparison of pretending at home. *Children Development, 70*, 1477–1488.
Kohlenberg, R. J., & Tsai, M. (1991). *Functional analytic psychotherapy: Creating intense and curative therapeutic relationships*. Plenum Press. https://doi.org/10.1007/978-0-387-70855-3
Krumboltz, J., & Krumboltz, H. (1977). *Modificação do comportamento infantil*. Editora EPU.
Leaper, C., & Smith, T. E. (2004). A meta-analytic review of gender variations in children's language use: Talkativeness, affiliative speech, and assertive speech. *Developmental Psychology, 40*, 993–1027.
Leaper, C., Anderson, K. J., & Sanders, P. (1998). Moderators of gender effects on parents' talk to their children: A meta-analysis. *Developmental Psychology, 34*, 3–27.
Moura, C. B., & Venturelli, M. B. (2004). Direcionamento para a Condução do Processo Terapêutico Comportamental com Crianças. *Revista Brasileira de Terapia Comportamental e Cognitiva, 6*, 17–30.
Oaklander, V. (1978). *Windows to our children: A gestalt approach to children and adolescents*. The Gestalt Journal Press.
Papalia, D. E., Olds, S. W., & Feldman, R. D. (2009). *Desenvolvimento humano*. McGraw-Hill.
Quintana, M. (2005). *Poesia completa*. Organização: Tania Franco Carvalhal. Nova Aguilar.

Rome-Flanders, T., Cronk, C., & Gourde, C. (1995). Maternal scaffolding in mother-infant games and its relationship to language development: A longitudinal study. *First Language, 15*, 339–355.

Skinner, B. F. (1953). *Science and human behavior*. Free Press.

Watson, T. S., & Gresham, F. M. (1998). *Handbook of child behavior therapy*. Plenum Press.

Chapter 8
Acceptance and Commitment Therapy: Interventions with Children

Aline Souza Simões, Raul Vaz Manzione, Desirée da Cruz Cassado, and Mônica Geraldi Valentim

Traditionally developed as a treatment for adult populations, acceptance and commitment therapy (ACT, read as one word ["ÁKT"/"ÉKT"] and not as an acronym) has been refined to fit children and youth audiences (Hayes & Greco, 2009; Hayes & Ciarrochi, 2015; McCurry & Hayes, 2009; Scarlet, 2017). ACT is inserted within the so-called contextual behavioral therapies, which have as philosophical paradigm the functional contextualism. This is a philosophical view of science similar to and, at the same time, distinct from radical behaviorism. The process of defining functional contextualism sets out to go beyond mere translation of radical behaviorist terms, proposing an important refinement in terms of extension and application.

Radical behaviorism is premised on the goal of predicting and controlling human behavior. According to Hayes (2019a), "'control' can refer to the elimination of variability, and the pragmatic goal of the contextual functional behavioral tradition is not to eliminate variability, but to make a difference" (p. 163). Therefore, a subtle change became necessary: control was replaced by influence, emphasizing the greater complexity of the behavior of human organisms compared to nonhuman organisms. Taking into account such complexity, functional contextualism uses relational framing theory (RFT) to address issues of human language and cognition.

The criterion of truth of contextualism is successful functioning: an analysis is considered true or valid as long as it leads to effective action, according to a certain objective. Thus, topographically mentalistic terms, hitherto rejected by the analytic-behavioral community, are now taken seriously if they enable – mediated by the functional-analytic gaze – an understanding of behavioral phenomena (Hayes,

---

A. S. Simões
Private Practice, Salvador, Brazil

R. V. Manzione (✉) · D. da Cruz Cassado
Private Practice, São Paulo, Brazil

M. G. Valentim
Ceconte - Brazilian Center for Contextual Behavior Science, São Paulo, Brazil

1984). Finally, models and theories based on evolutionary science and behavioral principles that facilitate the prediction and influence of behavior with accuracy, scope and depth are admitted – for example, the construction of the psychological flexibility model as an approach to psychopathology and its treatment and the development of Acceptance and Commitment Therapy (ACT) as an approach to the modification of psychological flexibility[1] of the realism controversy (as a philosophical debate) and enables the approach of behavioral issues in an analytical way, going according to the goals of contextual behavioral science.

ACT is presented as a multidimensional approach with a focus on reticulation, a model of scientific and practical development in which theoretical and technological progress occurs at multiple levels (functional contextualist philosophy, basic analytic-behavioral concepts, experimental research, applied research, intervention/public service provision) but in an interconnected way with different patterns of progress for the particular level of work. Thus, when "doing" ACT, one takes into account functional contextualism philosophy, basic behavioral concepts, and empirical research data (Baer et al., 1968; Hayes et al., 2012b; Westrup, 2014).

Because it is presented as a model, ACT is not, then, only an amalgamation of techniques and methods; its proposal is to promote psychological flexibility in different settings and populations. According to Hayes et al. (2012a, b), a unified model is a set of coherent processes that applies with precision, scope, and depth to a wide variety of clinically relevant problems and also applies to issues of human functioning and adaptability. The focus is not on the myriad of topographically defined forms of human suffering (symptoms and syndromes or symptom collective) but on the processes that have as their consequence the aforementioned suffering. This inflexibility is seen as a suffering-generating behavioral repertoire maintained by rigid rule-following (Hayes et al., 1999, 2012a, b).

Rule-Governed Behavior

From the moment we are born, we are exposed to environments where other human beings teach us how to use language. This is done initially by speaking to us, so that we become familiar with the sounds of that language. As development occurs, we are encouraged to produce similar sounds in our own way. Initially, these sounds are related to the world around us (e.g., "mommy," "daddy," "dog"). Quickly, we learn to relate such sounds to the private world: tastes, smells, feelings, sensations, and desires (e.g., "hunger," "thirst," "yummy," "disgusting," "pain," "want," "don't want," "yes," "no").

Around 14 to 16 months of age, language in human beings begins to differ from the language of other mammals (Hayes & Smith, 2005), and, around 23 months, they learn the behavior of deriving relations (Lipkens et al., 1993). The behavior of

---

[1] For an in-depth discussion, see Zettle et al. (2016) and Hayes (2019a, b).

deriving relations, unlike learning by direct contingencies, enables the learning of new relations between events without the obligation of exposure to situations (for example, imagine that Ana is hit by a toy tricycle, possibly resulting in a pain response. Later, Ana is told: "A car is **bigger than** the tricycle, **so be** careful." This enables Ana to learn to avoid contact with moving cars, because the probability of getting an aversive consequence is even greater).

ACT underpins its practice by *relational frame theory* (*RFT*), which explains the learning of the operant of deriving relations, mentioned above (relational arbitrarily applicable response (RRAA)). It is not up to this chapter, however, to address the emergence of RFT and its basic principles in depth[2], so only the most relevant aspects of this theory to be taken into account when addressing rule-governed behavior and psychopathology will be highlighted.

RFT states that during the period of language skill development, humans learn to relate arbitrary stimuli, which quickly becomes a generalized operant response through multiple exemplar training (exposure to multiple situations in which such an operant is emitted) (Healy et al., 2000). Through such multiple exemplar training, relational contextual cues (Crel[3], e.g., "same as," "opposite to," "greater than," "better than," and "part of") are abstracted and then applied arbitrarily to new stimuli.[4] The child will quickly be able to relate stimuli that don't share formal properties with each other. Thus, stimuli that have never been related in their learning history acquire functional properties; the functions to be established, however, depend on the social context that selects them (Luciano et al., 2009).

In an attempt to understand complex human behavior, Skinner (1966) proposed the concept of rules as antecedent stimuli that specify contingencies. Following rules, according to Skinner, enables the learning of new responses without the need for exposure to direct contingencies. From a view of RFT, it is said that rules alter the behavior of an individual through the transformation of functions resulting from contact with the elements included in them.

Rules are present in all contexts and periods of human development. Children delight in showing that they know the rules. At primary school age, they learn to behave according to the moment, for example, at playtime, or to sit in a chair and be quiet. By the end of primary school age, they know many rules that promote connection and cooperation. There are rules of behavior for different social contexts, for example, they learn to respond appropriately to the question, "How are you?"

There are three categories of rule-governed behaviors: *pliance*, *tracking*, and *augmenting*. *Pliance* is a category of verbally governed behavior[5] that happens under the influence of consequences that are mediated by a speaker. A child, about to go out to play, may hear his mother's rule: "Take a coat because it will be cold."

---

[2] See Barnes-Holmes et al. (2000), and Barnes-Holmes and O'Hora (2004).

[3] *Crel*: context in which a history of a particular type of relational responding is brought to bear on the current situation.

[4] "Arbitrary," here, refers to a type of stimulus that depends on social conventions.

[5] There is, as yet, no consensus on the official translation of the terms, so they are used in English.

In this example, the rule will be followed not because of the immediate consequence, since it is not cold at the moment, but because the mother, in the role of a talker, mediates the consequences of taking a coat (e.g., punishing if it is not done, gifting when it is done, etc.) (Hayes et al., 1989; Zettle & Hayes, 1982).

Tracking is behavior established by the verbal community once a certain level of behavior governed by *pliance* is present. It is a category of verbally governed behavior under the influence of the apparent correspondence of the rule and the way the environment is organized. For example, a child, after playing in the dirt and having dirty hands, may hear from an adult, "Let's wash your hands, because they are dirty." As the hands are washed, the child may be told that the hands are getting cleaner, without the addition of arbitrary social consequences for doing so. In this case, the consequence of washing hands is having clean hands (Hayes et al., 1989; Zettle & Hayes, 1982).

Augmenting is a type of rule that, instead of specifying consequences or contingencies (as is the case with *pliance* and *tracking*), modifies (increases) the reinforcing value of the consequences specified in the rule, having a similar function to motivational operations (Michael, 1993). In this case, for example, a child faced with a food he or she does not like (and therefore acting as an aversive antecedent stimulus) may hear from an adult, for example: "If you eat this, you will get big and strong!" If the rule is followed under the influence of adult-mediated consequences (e.g., approval), it may be considered *pliance*. If it is followed under the influence of the more delayed consequences of following (getting big and strong), it will be *augmenting*, because of the transformation from aversive to discriminative function. *Augmentals* may also specify consequences that are abstract and do not have to be directly contacted to exert control over behavior (e.g., development of morality and sense of justice) (Hayes et al., 1998; Carvalho, 2016).

Rules are not always helpful in promoting a prosperous life; verbal evaluations and rules tend to generate insensitivity to prevailing contingencies (Hayes, 1989). Imagine the hypothetical case of John, whose father abuses authority by belittling and assaulting him. It would be natural, therefore, for John to learn the rule: "adults cannot be trusted." In following it, it is possible that John – in coming into contact with other contexts, away from his father – misses important opportunities to develop trusting relationships with other adults, for example, with a kind teacher who wants to help him. The same complex human behavior (of following rules) that allows us to thrive as a species can also promote psychological inflexibility (Luciano & Hayes, 2001).

Psychological Flexibility and Inflexibility

The psychological flexibility model is by nature inductive and linked to basic human processes largely derived from basic science. It is a model of psychopathology, psychological well-being, and psychological intervention (Hayes et al., 2012a). Serving as a metaphor rather than the model itself, the six processes that contribute

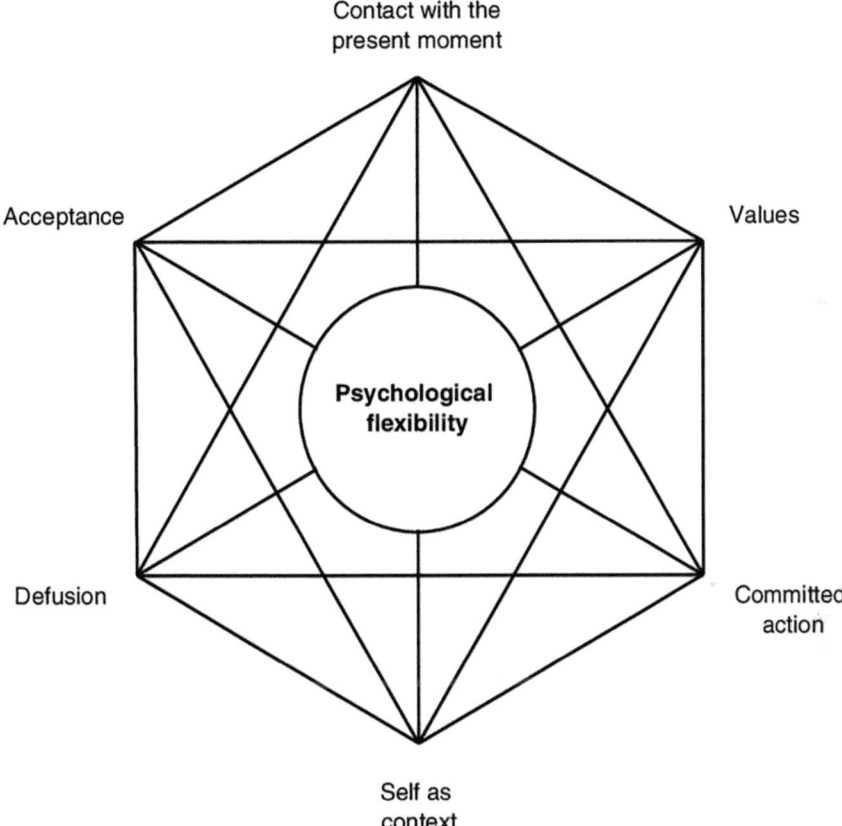

Fig. 8.1 Psychological inflexibility as a model of psychopathology

to psychological inflexibility are commonly represented in the figure of a hexagon[6] (Fig. 8.1), these being inflexible attention, disruption or lack of value clarity, inaction or impulsivity, attachment to concepts about the self, cognitive fusion, and experiential avoidance. In Fig. 8.2, the six core processes that correspond to psychological flexibility are presented: flexible attention to the present moment, chosen values, committed actions, self-with-context, defusion, and acceptance.

The four processes on the left (self-with-context, flexible attention to the present moment, acceptance, and defusion) refer to *mindfulness* and acceptance processes; the four processes on the right (self-with-context, flexible attention to the present moment, committed action, and values) are commitment and behavioral activation/behavioral change processes. The processes of self-within-context and flexible attention to the present moment are present in both.

---

[6] Just as a way of representing the processes of psychological flexibility, this hexagon is nicknamed "hexaflex" – that is, a hexagon representing psychological flexibility.

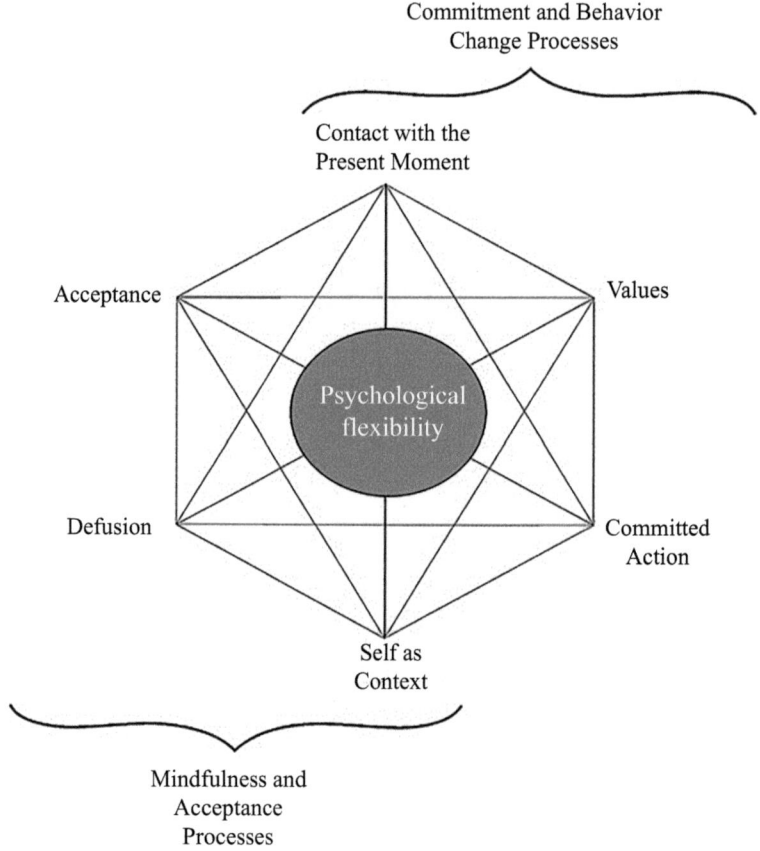

Fig. 8.2 Psychological flexibility as a human model of functioning and behavioral change

Psychological flexibility, thus defined, would be the behavioral repertoire that makes the individual able to contact the present moment as a conscious human being, in an integral manner, divesting himself of unnecessary defenses. In this situation, he is capable of interpreting the situation as it presents itself and not as it appears. Based on what the situation allows, it is the gesture of persisting or changing behavior, in the service of chosen values (Hayes et al., 2012a, b). It is a model that assumes that the core of psychopathology and human suffering is psychological inflexibility, consisting of attempts to control psychological reactions to discomfort when they compromise the possibility of engaging in value-based actions.

Despite being a fairly new approach within psychology, at the time of writing, there are 296 randomized clinical trials on the subject, and this number is still expanding (Hayes, 2019b). Although there are considerably fewer empirical studies with children, significant growth in interest in the utility of ACT in this population is observed. A review study (Swain et al., 2015) concluded that emerging research is encouraging in this regard. In recent years, ACT has increasingly established itself as a transdiagnostic model[7]. Alternatively, unified or transdiagnostic treatment protocols have been put forward to address different diagnostic categories, focusing on core features of disorders. Many disorders defined in the Diagnostic and Statistical Manual of Mental Disorders[8] share common dimensions such as impulse control difficulties, attentional control problems, rumination or preoccupation, cognitive inflexibility, and self-awareness difficulties, among others.

The goal of the most modern behavioral and cognitive therapies is not to eliminate, modify, or suppress private events (feelings, thoughts, sensations, and memories) but to promote more positive life trajectories. To do so, it is necessary to know the processes that foster growth and development so that more effective interventions can be developed (Hayes & Hoffman, 2018). Therefore, from a process-based therapy perspective, thinking about children's ACT involves thinking about processes shared by this population and how to adapt interventions so that they are accessible to different levels of development.

ACT for Children

Given that ACT focuses on language-derived processes, working with children is of particular importance. Studies show that the issues of concern to children of varying ages have a recognizable pattern: the older the child, the greater the complexity and variety of their concerns (e.g., Chorpita et al., 1997). This statement may seem simple at first glance, but it touches on the issue that has a central place in discussions in ACT and RFT: language development. The more developed a child's language processes, the greater and more complex their concerns (e.g., Vasey & Daleiden, 1994).

When we work with the common focus of ACT, typically developing adults, we are dealing with individuals whose language processes are refined and complex and whose behavior, therefore, is under a great deal of verbal control. ACT processes are then intended to minimize this control and to give the subject tools to live the life they would like to live. An important reflection, therefore, and one that has been increasingly discussed is: what is the impact of these tools for an audience whose language control is still in its early stages of development?

In early childhood, children respond to stimuli that are present in the immediate environment, and their behavior is governed by the direct consequences of their behavior (Greco et al., 2005). Thus, for example, for a child, the behavior of touching a dog may decrease in frequency after a bite, and the probability of vocalizing the word "mommy" may increase if it is followed by gestures of attention and affection.

---

[7] That applies to more than one condition.
[8] 5th edition; DSM-5 (American Psychiatric Association, 2013).

However, as children grow older, their behavior becomes under control not only of direct contingencies but also of verbal contingencies (Greco et al., 2005). Thus, we can imagine the following situation: Pedro was bitten by a dog when he was little and, since then, has fearful reactions and moves away when he sees any dog (dogs in general acquire an aversive function through the generalization process). At school, he hears a friend telling him that he hates cats, because a cat scratched him, and that they are much worse than dogs. In this situation, Peter's avoidance and evasion behaviors toward cats may increase in frequency. Although he has never suffered any negative consequences from direct contact with a cat, the history of verbal learning related to the contextual cue "worse than" influences the stimulus "cat" to stop being neutral and start acquiring aversive functions enhanced by its relation with the stimulus "dog."

From situations like Peter's, verbal individuals also begin to behave under control of consequences that exist only in language. As they grow up, children respond more and more to verbal stimuli, and rules about past, present, and future increasingly influence their behavior. Studies linking childhood anxiety and overprotective parents (e.g., Greco & Morris, 2002; Rapee, 1997; Rapee & Melville, 1997), for example, suggest that a child who has grown up in a context where he or she constantly heard rules about care and protection may follow rules derived from these, in which the world takes on an aversive function, as a dangerous place. Thus, even stimuli usually considered neutral can be seen as aversive, as well as feelings and thoughts related to these experiences.

With the aim of weakening the control of rules that restrict the subject's behavior and strengthening a value-directed repertoire (i.e., psychological flexibility), ACT proposes interventions in six fields: acceptance, cognitive defusion, *self-with-context*, present moment contact, values, and committed action (Hayes et al., 2012a, b). Interventions in each of the fields involve, in addition to analytic interventions (i.e., molar and molecular functional analysis), strategies such as experiential exercises and metaphors, which are useful tools in providing context for less rigid language use. Through strategies like this, therefore, ACT aims at a change of context, which will alter the individual's relationship with the relational response itself (Hayes et al., 2012a, b). Thus, the child inserted in the overprotective context, for example, can, in therapy, learn to respond to his own feelings and thoughts about possible threats, looking at them from a flexible perspective, with the possibility of relating to them in different ways.

Such strategies, if considered in the context of child therapy, may facilitate the communication and engagement of children and adolescents, since they escape a purely discursive therapeutic context. Based on the assumptions of functional contextualism, the child therapist can formulate the case conceptualization and understand the function of his/her client's repertoire, having the flexibility to use strategies already presented in the ACT literature, as well as to formulate play interventions that are useful for each case. To illustrate this process, we will discuss the field of cognitive defusion, a component of hexaflex. Cognitive defusion consists of responding to private stimuli (feelings, sensations, thoughts) as what they are (i.e., feelings, sensations, and thoughts), rather than responding to them as fact or reality (Hayes et al., 2012a, b). Consider, then, that 10-year-old Isabela, after her parents' separation, is faced with constant thoughts that she needs to take care of her mother or something horrible will happen to her. When Isabela cries and fights with her mother so she won't leave or won't accept being alone at her father's house, we can say that she is responding to the content of her thoughts. If the mother responds to the child's behavior, by not going out, for example, we can say that the probability of occurrence of that behavior increases from the process of negative reinforcement.

A therapist who understands this dynamic could work with Isabella on ways to change the context in which that thought arises and transform its functions. One strategy for cognitive defusion might be to write or draw the thoughts on a whiteboard in different ways. Meanwhile, therapist and client are talking about the thoughts as clouds in the sky that come and go. Here the therapist tries to model with the child the behavior of looking at the thought and responding to it for what it really is: just a thought, without having to act to avoid or modify it (connecting to the field of acceptance). Another aspect to be considered in psychotherapeutic work with children is the inclusion of the family in the process. Considering that parents or caregivers are usually the most significant part of the child's context, their inclusion is necessary in most of the sessions. Interventions in this sense include aspects commonly covered by traditional behavior analytic therapy, such as psychoeducation, guidance, and functional analysis of family dynamics. When considering the problematic worked by ACT, it is necessary to reflect on the importance of analyzing how the six aspects of psychological inflexibility worked by hexaflex also present themselves in the family (Coyne et al., 2011; Swain et al., 2015).

The adults who play a central role in the child's life mostly come from an advanced process of language development and rule-following. The central phenomenon of ACT, experiential avoidance, is commonly evident in the caregiver who brings the child to therapy. Considering the cultural context in which the normal is to feel good and suffering should be avoided, the adult may engage in avoidance and evasion behaviors of their own aversive private events arising from contact with the child's different forms of suffering. Through modelling and shaping processes, the child often comes to the clinic presenting a rigid behavioral pattern of experiential avoidance which is also a reflection of the caregiver's way of dealing with his/her private events (Greco et al., 2005).

From the ACT perspective, a possible path would be to work the fields of psychological flexibility also through interventions with caregivers and child together. In this way, the cognitive defusion exercise mentioned earlier could be done with the adult present, also talking about his own private events and building, together with the child, new ways to respond to them.

ACT is a model that, even in its work with adults, uses experiential, playful, and not very literal interventions with the aim of weakening the control exercised by language. For children, developing individuals, this kind of intervention can be even richer and bring a new range of possibilities. Here the therapist finds a unique opportunity: working less to remedy problems generated by language and more to prevent them, contributing to the formation of subjects capable of dealing with their own suffering more effectively and thus able to walk toward what makes life worth living.

References

American Psychiatric Association. (2013). *Diagnostic and statistical manual of mental disorders* (5th ed.) https://doi-org.ezproxy.frederick.edu/10.1176/appi.books.9780890425596

Baer, D. M., Wolf, M. M., & Risley, T. R. (1968). Some current dimensions of applied behavior analysis. *Journal of Applied Behavior Analysis, 1*, 91–97.

Barnes-Holmes, D., & O'Hora, D. (2004). Instructional control: Developing a relational frame analysis. *International Journal of Psychology and Psychological Therapy, 4*, 263–284.

Barnes-Holmes, D., Barnes-Holmes, Y., & Cullinan, V. (2000). Relational frame theory and Skinner's verbal behavior: A possible synthesis. *The Behavior Analyst, 23*, 69–84.

Carvalho, L. M. (2016). *Desenvolvimento moral na Análise do Comportamento: uma revisão bibliográfica*. Dissertação de Mestrado. Instituto de Psicologia, Universidade de São Paulo.

Chorpita, B. F., Tracey, S. A., Brown, T. A., Collica, T. J., & Barlow, D. H. (1997). Assessment of worry in children and adolescents: An adaptation of the Penn State Worry Questionnaire. *Behaviour Research and Therapy, 35*, 569–581.

Coyne, L., Mchugh, L., & Evan, R. M. (2011). Acceptance and commitment therapy (ACT): Advances and applications with children, adolescents, and families. *Child and Adolescent Psychiatric Clinics of North America, 20*, 379–399.

Greco, L., & Hayes, S. C. (2009). *Acceptance and mindfulness treatments for children and adolescents: A practitioner's guide*. New Harbinger Publications.

Greco, L. A., & Morris, T. L. (2002). Paternal child-rearing style and child social anxiety: Investigation of child perceptions and actual father behavior. *Journal of Psychopathology and Behavioral Assessment, 24*, 259–267.

Greco, L. A., Blackledge, J. T., Coyne, L. W., & Enreheich, J. (2005). Integrating acceptance and mindfulness into treatments for child and adolescent anxiety disorders: Acceptance and commitment therapy as an example. In S. M. Orsillo & L. Roemer (Eds.), *Acceptance and mindfulness-based approaches to anxiety: Conceptualization and treatment*. Kluwer/Plenum.

Hayes, S. C. (1984). Making sense of spirituality. *Behavior, 12*, 99–110.

Hayes, S. C. (Org.). (1989). *Rule-governed behavior: Cognition, contingencies and instructional control*. Plenum Press.

Hayes, S. C. (2019a). *ACT randomized controlled trials since 1986*. https://contextualscience.org/ACT_Randomized_Controlled_Trials

Hayes, S. C. (2019b). Ciência Comportamental Contextual. In D. Zilio & K. Carrara (Eds.), *Behaviorismos: Reflexões Históricas e Conceituais* (Vol. 3). Editora Paradigma.

Hayes, L., & Ciarrochi, L. (2015). *The thriving adolescent: Using acceptance and commitment therapy and positive psychology to help teens manage emotions, achieve goals, and build connection*. New Harbinger Publications.

Hayes, S. C., & Hoffman, S. (2018). *Process-based CBT: The science and core clinical competencies of cognitive behavioral therapy*. New Harbinger Publications.

Hayes, S. C., & Smith, S. (2005). *Get out of your mind and into your life: Thenew acceptance and commitment therapy*. New Harbinger.

Hayes, S. C., Zettle, R. D., & Rosenfarb, I. (1989). Rule following. In: S. C. Hayes (Org.), *Rule-governed behavior: Cognition, contingencies, and instructional control* (pp. 191–220). Plenum.

Hayes, S. C., Gifford, E. V., & Hayes, G. J. (1998). Moral behavior and the development of verbal regulation. *The Behavior Analyst, 21*(2), 253–279.

Hayes, S. C., Strosahl, K., & Wilson, K. (1999). *Acceptance and commitment. Therapy: An experiential approach to behavior change*. The Guilford Press.

Hayes, S. C., Barnes-Holmes, D., & Wilson, K. (2012a). Contextual behavioral science: Creating a science more adequate to the challenge of the human condition. *Journal of Contextual Behavioral Science*. https://doi.org/10.1016/j.jcbs.2012.09.004

Hayes, S. C., Strosahl, K., & Wilson, K. (2012b). *Acceptance and commitment therapy: The process and practice of mindful change*. The Guilford Press.

Healy, O., Barnes-Holmes, D., & Smeets, P. M. (2000). Derived relational responding as generalized operant behavior. *Journal of the Experimental Analysis of Behavior, 74*(2), 207–227.

Lipkens, G., Hayes, S. C., & Hayes, L. J. (1993). Longitudinal study of derived stimulus relations in an infant. *Journal of Experimental Child Psychology, 56*, 201–239.

Luciano, C., & Hayes, S. C. (2001). Trastorno de Evitación Experiencial. *Revista Internacional de Psicología Clínica y de la Salud, 1*, 109–157.

Luciano, C., Valdivia-Salas, S., Cabello, F., & Hernández, M. (2009). Developing self-directed rules. In R. A. Rehfeldt & Y. Barnes-Holmes (Eds.), *Derived relational responding. Applications for learners with autism and other developmental disabilities* (pp. 335–352). New Harbinger Publications.

McCurry, C., & Hayes, S. C. (2009). *Parenting your anxious child with mindfulness and acceptance: A powerful new approach to overcoming fear, panic, and worry using acceptance and commitment therapy*. New Harbinger Publications.

Michael, J. (1993). Establishing operations. *The Behavior Analyst, 16*(2), 191–206.

Rapee, R. M. (1997). Potential role of childrearing practices in the development of anxiety and depression. *Clinical Psychology Review, 17*, 47–67.

Rapee, R. M., & Melville, L. F. (1997). Recall of family factors in social phobia and panic disorder: Comparison of mother and offspring reports. *Depression and Anxiety, 5*, 7–11.

Scarlet, S. (2017). Superhero therapy: A hero's journey through acceptance and commitment therapy. .

Skinner, B. F. (1966). An operant analysis of problem solving. In B. Kleinmuntz (Ed.), *Problem solving: Research, method and theory*. Wiley.

Swain, J., Hancock, K., Dixon, A., & Bowman, J. (2015). Acceptance and commitment therapy for children: A systematic review of intervention studies. *Journal of Contextual Behavioral Science, 4*(2), 73–85.

Vasey, M. W., & Daleiden, E. L. (1994). Worry in children. In G. Davey & F. Tallis (Eds.), *Worrying: Perspectives on theory, assessment, and treatment* (pp. 185–207). Wiley.

Westrup, D. (2014). *Advanced acceptance and commitment therapy: The experienced Practitioner's guide to optimizing delivery*. New Harbinger Publications.

Zettle, R. D., & Hayes, S. C. (1982). Rule governed behavior: A potential theoretical framework for cognitive behavior therapy. In P. C. Kendall (Ed.), *Advances in cognitive behavioral research and therapy* (pp. 73–118). Academic.

Zettle, R. D., et al. (2016). *The Wiley handbook of contextual Behavioral science*. Wiley.

Chapter 9
Introduction to Functional-Analytic Psychotherapy with Children

Cynthia Borges de Moura

Introduction to Functional-Analytic Psychotherapy with Children

Behavior therapy changed its focus significantly after some therapist-researchers took the risk of applying the Skinnerian model to the clinical context. Although Skinner was not a therapist and was not specifically concerned with clinical problems, the theoretical and philosophical assumptions that he introduced within the scope of scientific behavior analysis led behavioral therapists to a new understanding and intervention with their clients. Several aspects of the Skinnerian approach, for example, the recognition of the value of self-observation, the analysis of private events, and the proposition of a functional analysis of verbal behavior and its influence on other behaviors, contributed to the overcoming of mentalistic proposals and to the construction of a truly behaviorist identity for behavioral therapy.

In the 1980s, two different groups of researchers led by Hayes (1987) and Kohlenberg and Tsai (1987) developed models of clinical intervention with adults from the perspective indicated by Skinner's radical behaviorism, which took shape in the 2000s (Hayes, 2004; Kohlenberg & Tsai, 1991). These models, in general, have been applied to clinical problems by providing a language and a conceptualization concerning human nature and the interaction between an individual's behavior and the natural environment. Although they follow different paths in strategic terms, both have congruent therapeutic goals. Hayes adopts an approach that aims to intervene on the control of behavior as a way to obtain the alteration of the client's specific problem. Kohlenberg takes the problem behavior itself as the unit and starting point for a comprehensive and broad functional analysis. Since the behavior

---

C. B. de Moura (✉)
Instituto Terapia Criativa, Universidade Estadual do Oeste do Paraná,
Foz do Iguaçu, PR, Brazil

occurs in the clinical context, the therapeutic relationship is seen as the appropriate instance to bring about the desired changes.

Functional-analytic psychotherapy (FAP), proposed by Kohlenberg and Tsai (1987, 1991), is part of what has been called third wave or third-generation therapies (Hayes, 2004; Pérez Álvarez, 2006). And, as such, it shares with other therapies of this generation the applications of advances in the study of behavior: the equivalence relations between stimuli, the behavior governed by rules, the functional analysis of verbal behavior, and its impact on understanding cognition and emotions (Fernández Parra & Ferro García, 2006).

According to Hayes (2004), what characterizes the third wave therapies is the greater attention to the context and functions of psychological phenomena and not only to their form. Therefore, they tend to propose contextual and experiential change strategies in addition to classical didactic strategies. These are treatments that seek, together with the client, to build a broad, flexible, assertive, and effective behavioral repertoire rather than a specific approach to narrowly defined problems. In short, third wave therapies focus on the way language affects experience, the therapeutic relationship, the concept of mindfulness, the self as context, and acceptance.

Although it was not designed for clinical practice with children, the FAP proposal seems to be well suited to the context of child psychotherapy (Moura & Conte, 1997). In the rest of this chapter, I analyzed how, from a certain point of view, the proposal of Kohlenberg and Tsai (1991) can be used in clinical practice with children and, in this way, also legitimize a radical behaviorist action of the child behavioral therapist. Although we consider the action of the child therapist with parents or carers fundamental, we will purposely exclude the discussion in this sense, since the purpose of this chapter is to specifically approach the FAP with children.

The FAP Model Extended to Therapy with Children

The FAP approach is based largely on a proposal to apply procedures based on the principles of behavior analysis within the limits of the typical clinical treatment context. One of these limits is established by the fact that the therapist-client contact is generally restricted to the moment of therapy, and it is difficult or almost impossible for the therapist to observe and interact with the client outside the session.

However, what is configured as a limit can also be an opportunity for significant changes from the intimate and intense relationship established between therapist and client, which offers the client a live learning setting, helping him to deal with the problem in the here and now and, thus, acquire skills to overcome his problems in daily life.

These conditions also apply to the context of child psychotherapy, because we hardly have access to the child outside the clinical context for some kind of intervention and, because he/she is a child, the relationship with him/her is also hardly distant or impersonal. Thus, given that the child audience "fits" the FAP proposal, mainly because children's therapy works a lot with direct modeling, it becomes relevant to consider how the central characteristics of the approach of Kohlenberg and Tsai (1991) can be applied to work with them in order to intensify the possible results of the psychotherapeutic process.

The Use of Reinforcement

Reinforcement in the clinical context plays an important role in the FAP model, since the main aspect of behavioral-analytic treatment is direct modeling through differential reinforcement of required repertoires during therapy sessions. A well-known aspect of reinforcement is that the closer in time and space the behavior is in relation to its consequences, the greater the control exerted by them. This concept is fundamental to the work of the child behavior therapist, because in the session, as the interaction with the therapist takes place, based on the planned intervention, the therapist can model and strengthen the child's behaviors, desirable for overcoming his problems. When the same behaviors occur at home or at school, far from the therapist's direct observation, modeling becomes the responsibility of parents or teachers, not always sufficiently prepared for the task.

With the identification of the probable contingencies present in the natural environment, from the child's report or representation (drawings, stories, games, make-believe games), the therapist can act in an alternative way, confronting the child with a new way of understanding or dealing with the situation, thus weakening possible distorted perceptions and fanciful relations between events, giving the child the opportunity to experience new interactions that produce behavioral changes and emotional growth.

The child psychotherapist may have many artificial resources for reinforcement, such as rewarding the achievement of a certain behavioral criterion in the session, with colored stickers or access to a "secret," such as learning a magic trick, for example. Kohlenberg and Tsai (1991), however, point out that natural reinforcers, that is, spontaneous actions and reactions between client and therapist, are usually potentially more powerful in generating significant change. In the natural environment, the spontaneous expressions of people involved in an interaction are reinforced by the reciprocal positive responsiveness between them. Thus, for example, if the child's expression of affection is a target behavior and the therapist also has a spontaneously affectionate reaction when she emits it, the reinforcement will most likely be natural, which favors behavioral generalization in this direction.

Arbitrary reinforcement, however, can be useful as a transitional procedure in child therapy. It can increase sensitivity to environmental stimuli more quickly and make it easier for the therapist to conduct more concrete analyses of the child's own behavior. On the other hand, arbitrary reinforcement can also replace or interfere with the possibility that natural reinforcers gain control over behavior (Ferster, 1979). For this reason, they should be used sparingly, although experience shows that, in general, children "dismiss" arbitrary stimuli, as if they no longer made sense when compared to naturally reinforcing consequences inherent to the behavior.

Clinically Relevant Behaviors (CRBs) and the Clinical Environment as an Agent of Change

Kohlenberg and Tsai's (1991) model is also characterized by its attention to the specification of behaviors of interest. The term "clinically relevant behavior" (CRB) includes both problem behavior and target behavior. Thus, the child psychotherapist needs to be a skilled observer, because careful clinical observations are the basis for defining CRBs. Obviously, the child's problem behavior cannot be directly observed unless it happens in the therapist's presence, even if the therapist can obtain a good description through the parents' or other observers' report or can watch it through a videotape recording. Thus, the therapeutic environment will be considered adequate for promoting direct changes if the problem behaviors presented by the child are of such a nature that they can also occur during the session. Based on this criterion, the functional-analytic approach focuses on problems of the outside world that also occur during the session, which does not mean that it is not also possible to deal with those that do not occur, such as enuresis, for example.

The applicability of this aspect to child behavior therapy needs to be well understood, because the problems that children present may occur in the session, both directly, in the therapist-child relationship, and indirectly, in the way they behave during the proposed playful situations. Thus, a child with complaints of aggressiveness, for example, does not necessarily need to attack the therapist in order for him to deal with the problem (in fact, it is more comfortable if this does not occur, although it may eventually happen) but may demonstrate this pattern of conduct through story characters or a toy situation.

The play or story may show the therapist the contingencies that established the child's aggressive behavior and provide a good opportunity to investigate its current function. During this analysis, the therapist may also discuss with the child the alternatives for more socially appropriate behavior of the character, request the emission of more cooperative behavior in the game, or discuss the similarities between the behavior of the character in the story and his own or between the behavior emitted in the game and the behavior with friends at school (Conte & Regra, 2000; Moura & Conte, 1997). This information will also serve as important subsidies for guidance to parents and other adults of interest.

The selection and discriminability of CRBs by the child therapist will be facilitated if he/she has developed, in his/her personal repertoire, the target behaviors he/she wants to achieve with the child. This seems obvious because the therapist is an adult and the client is a child, but in practice it is not. It means having developed in yourself skills considered appropriate and been able to observe similar reactions in the child, such as remaining relaxed, knowing how to play and have fun, knowing how to deal with frustration and defeat, and dealing with demands and pressure. They also need to have the ability to do things that children like, be flexible and creative, and not be anxious about obtaining immediate positive results (Conte, 1993). These characteristics of the therapist will help the child to adapt more easily and quickly to the clinical environment and to present his most typical and "natural" reactions. Importantly, when observing and assessing the appropriateness of the child's behavior, the therapist should be sensitive to the child's level of development and to the characteristics of the current context and social environment in which the child lives.

According to Kohlenberg and Tsai (1991), a factor that restricts the range of target behaviors selected in a traditional therapy is the requirement that these refer only to the observable. They state that, in practice, it is almost impossible to achieve such objectivity when faced with applied problems, that inferences are not only necessary but useful. In many moments, the therapist needs to use his own "personal impressions" to raise hypotheses and verify the functionality of certain behaviors. This applies to the child therapist as well. The FAP therapist intervenes by testing his hypotheses: if they are confirmed, his acting strategies can be maintained; otherwise, others should be implemented. The important thing is that the professional is guided and reinforced by the client's improvements and progress, also outside the clinical environment.

Traditionally, the best way to create conditions for the generalization of the progress obtained by the client would be to conduct therapy in the same environment where the problem occurs. In Kohlenberg and Tsai's (1991) view, this is not necessary, as there is a functional similarity between the therapeutic context and the client's daily environment and clinically relevant behaviors tend to occur in both. This concept radically changes the child behavior therapist's practice, as he can, through his relationship with the child, directly evaluate the occurrence of both problems and improvements and thus favor the generalization of progress.

In summary, the most important characteristic of a problem that makes it suitable for child FAP is the possibility of its occurrence during the therapy session. This conclusion is based on the following assumptions: (1) the specific effects of therapy result from events that happen during the session, and the only controlling events that can happen at that time are discriminative – therapist can function as a discriminative stimulus for a situation in which certain client behaviors are more likely to occur; eliciters – therapist can evoke client emotional responses, sensations, images, or thoughts; or reinforcers – therapist reacts in ways that increase the occurrence of certain client behaviors; (2) occurring within the session, these events will have greater effects on behavior occurring in the same environment, so improvements may be naturally reinforced by contingencies provided by the therapist or conditions arranged in therapy.

The CRBs of Children in the Process of Therapy

Live learning opportunities emerge in the therapeutic relationship when the client emits clinically relevant behaviors in relation to the therapist's person. These are moments when behavior can be modeled directly from the effects on the relationship. Kohlenberg and Tsai (1991) describe three types of client behavior that may occur during the session, of particular relevance to the therapeutic process. In this sense, although the whole description refers to the clinical context with adults, children seem to demonstrate more clearly during sessions the clinically relevant behaviors with which you can work.

CRB1 refers to instances of behavior that happen during the therapy session that are occurrences of the clinical problem. These behaviors should decrease in frequency during the course of therapy. CRB1s usually consist of avoidance behaviors that, in the client's daily life, are under the control of aversive stimuli, which are often accompanied by negative emotional states. A child's rude behavior in answering her questions may be both proximity avoidance, due to negative experiences with attachment figures, and a resistance to yielding to her control, due to a history of "being obeyed" by the adults in her environment.

Children may come to therapy with low self-esteem and a low sense of competence, showing dislike for themselves, not feeling able to achieve or recognize success and social approval in their accomplishments. Or they may arrive with apparently "high" self-esteem, also hiding a sense of social or academic incompetence. In any case, they will relate to the therapist in the way they relate to other people and will provide samples of the problems to be worked on.

Here are some examples of behaviors to be observed: does the child look at you, greet you, and smile? Does he/she enter without the mother, or does he/she enter with the mother and accepts to stay without her? Does the child follow your instructions or ignore your commands? Does the child look around and pick up objects or walk around the room? Does he/she talk like a baby? Does he/she make a point of cooperating or contradicting? Is he pushy, agitated, difficult to remain seated? Stubborn, knocks things over? Concerned with organization or cleanliness? Impatient, irritable, short tempered? Does he/she bite fingernails? Keeps hand or fingers in mouth? Refuses to try a game/activity that he/she does not know or chosen by you? Is shy, timid, soft-spoken, monosyllabic?

Children often use indirect communication through play, drawings, and stories to demonstrate their feelings and other related behaviors, such as their perception of the environment. These are rich opportunities for observation and identification of CRBs1. They may frown after losing a single game, draw tiny pictures in a corner of the paper, tear up their drawing and throw it in the trash (or tear up their drawing!), model a family of snakes with play dough, or model a cage with the whole family inside.

When the therapist participates in the fantasy and, through it, provides opportunities for children to experience new experiences indirectly, they tend to gradually acquire greater self-control and begin to communicate more directly. By acting this way, the therapist provides the child with the feeling of being understood and supported and thus creates a less aversive context for the development of the child's ability to recognize, analyze, and change problematic behaviors and feelings, paving the way for more adapted behavioral solutions, which, according to FAP, constitute the CRB2s.

CRB2 refers to those repertoires whose absence or low strength are directly related to the present problem. These behaviors must increase in strength during the course of treatment to indicate progress or improvement. During the early stages of treatment, these repertoires are usually not observed, probably due to the lack of experiences in their natural environment that could have favored the development of these types of behavior. Possible CRB2s include assertive behavioral repertoires, positive emotional expressiveness, appropriate problem-solving, higher self-esteem, and a greater sense of competence, among others.

Let us return to the hypothetical situation of the child who presented a rude response to the therapist's questions and proposals for activities, as a proximity dodge. Now she responds without rudeness, draws a picture to give to the therapist, hugs him on the way out, and spontaneously tells facts about her week. Or, for example, the child who was always obeyed accepts to play "follow the boss," asks (not tells!) to do some specific activity, accepts to wait when the therapist tells him they will do it the following week. These are small changes in the desired direction, modeled very probably by the reinforcing characteristics of interaction with the therapist, who reciprocally responds to pro-social behavior and affective interaction. Another example is the child who "doesn't remember" what happened when the therapist approaches him about occurrences of the problem behavior during the week. When he realizes that he will not be punished in this environment, he begins to "remember," reports such occurrences more spontaneously, and accepts your suggestions for alternative solutions.

Progressively, the child begins to use more direct verbal communication in therapy, using more of the "I" and less of the "fantasy character." At this point, more directive interventions and strategies can gradually be introduced. When the child becomes more aware of his open and covert behavioral patterns, he will be able to produce changes in his environment, collaborating with the efforts of the responsible adults. Experience has shown that modeling and reinforcing the CRB2s during the session favors the generalization of therapeutic gains to situations outside the clinic, by the same principle of functional similarity.

As a result of the previous step, CRB3 is constituted by children's verbalizations about the correspondence between CRBs 1 and 2 and their controlling variables. It refers to children talking about their own behavior and what seems to cause it. More specifically, this involves the observation of the behavior itself and the associated reinforcing, discriminative, and eliciting stimuli. This description of functional relationships can help the child make generalization of their progress and obtain reinforcement in daily life. According to Kohlenberg and Tsai (1991), CRB3 repertoires also include descriptions of functional equivalences that indicate similarities between the situation-stimulus present during the session and those occurring outside the treatment.

According to this definition, developing CRB3 seems a big, or even impossible, task for children. Experience has shown that, on the contrary, respected the limits of their development, children discover this reasoning and use it in a special and useful way. For example, one of the author's patients, 8 years old, practically "fought" with her because of an attentional training with the use of Sudoku on the cell phone. As he presented some difficulty, he refused and wanted to give up in the middle. In one of the sessions when he was close to finishing and the therapist held him in the activity for him to finish it, he left angry saying "I hate you and your Chinese puzzle!" But the next session, surprisingly, he asked to do it again and did much better. The therapist celebrated the effort and praised the initiative, as well as the result, and ended by saying "we even fought about it last week, remember? It was ugly what I did, do you forgive me? You were just teaching me something that I have to do at school too, wasn't it? Now I've learned that I can do it".

It is not always possible, however, for therapists to observe the achievement of this stage, not because the children are not capable but because, when progress starts to occur, many parents interrupt the therapy, for feeling satisfied with the partial results obtained or bothered with the increase in the child's autonomy, expressiveness, and assertiveness (Moura & Conte, 1997). However, the achievement of such goal may figure as a discharge criterion in child therapy, since it impacts the child's global development.

The Skills of the Functional-Analytic Child Psychotherapist

The assessment procedures in FAP to generate clinical hypotheses and monitor the client's progress are the same used by other child therapists: interviews, self-reports, questionnaires, records, drawings, stories, and games. Throughout the treatment, however, he interacts honestly with the child, expressing his feelings to her and her behaviors in order to intensify the therapeutic relationship and make the therapeutic setting a place of genuine learning.

Given that psychotherapy is a complex interactional process involving multidetermined behaviors, Kohlenberg and Tsai (1991) suggest some rules for the therapist's behavior, which, according to them, if followed, result in reinforcing effects. The first rule prescribes the development of a good observation repertoire, as a prerequisite for the therapist to identify possible instances of CRBs occurring during the session and, thus, to react appropriately and consistently to them. Observation can increase the likelihood that progress will be reinforced and inappropriate behaviors extinguished or punished.

The second rule is widely used by child psychotherapists: building a therapeutic environment favorable to the evocation of CRBs. With children, it is not possible to work only at the verbal level, and it becomes necessary to use the playful language, proper of children. According to Conte (1993), when attending children, the therapist should explore the behavior of playing through strategies that interest them, such as drawings, comics, storybooks, painting, music, and other playful resources, as a form of metaphorical expression of the child about his relations with the world and his public and private reactions. Play helps to make explicit to the child the antecedent and consequent situations of their responses and to identify the occurrence of similar behaviors inside and outside the session, as well as to raise with the child more adaptive alternatives to the problem they face and to train new skills.

The third rule calls the therapist's attention to the value of immediate positive reinforcement of CRB2s. If problem behaviors can be detected and worked on within the clinical situation itself, it is assumed that improvements can and should also take place within the session and thus be valued and strengthened by the therapist. For reinforcement to occur appropriately, the therapist must be clear which incompatible behavior should be reinforced so that he/she can then be sensitive to small behavioral changes towards the desired improvement. When the child begins to abandon his inadequate behavior patterns; to present a more positive interaction with the therapist, significant others, and his environment; and to develop more appropriate problem-solving alternatives, it is time to value such progress and feel reinforced by it.

Being able to naturally reinforce the client's improvements by feeling reinforced by them is an important therapeutic skill, and, to help therapists acquire it, Kohlenberg and Tsai (1991) proposed a fourth rule: it is important that the therapist develop a repertoire of observation of the potentially reinforcing properties of his or her behavior, contingent on the occurrences of the client's clinically relevant behavior. This rule, basically, prescribes a good repertoire of self-awareness and self-observation for the therapist, so that he/she can discriminate during the therapeutic process which of his/her reactions evoke the child's problem behavior and which reinforce the development of the target behaviors.

Thus, during the consultations, I adopted the practice of playing, saying that I will "faint with emotion" when they achieve something difficult. Depending on the child's reaction to the first use of the joke, we can tell if it will have a reinforcing effect or not: some children look at me with a face of "that's not funny," and others burst out laughing and ask to see another fainting spell. The fourth rule increases the therapist's discrimination regarding the therapeutic function of his personal resources, always keeping in mind that a reinforcing relationship with his client is fundamental to the process.

The fifth rule emphasizes the development of a repertoire of description of functional relations between the controlling variables and the child's behavior, a priority for good therapeutic performance, because it would be incongruous to intervene and try to help the other to develop self-awareness when one does not understand the interrelations and determinations of the behavior in focus. For the 8-year-old Sudoku fighting client reported earlier, my response was: "Wow, you achieved two difficult things: doing Sudoku in record time and finding out why we are training to do difficult things!"

This is a simplified response to the child. Behind the scenes, the therapist needs to understand the more complex relationships established between the child and his/her family, school members, friends, and agents of other social institutions. In this case, why does a child cry and stop trying to complete his activities at school at the slightest sign of difficulty? How did the family install this behavior protecting the child from bigger problems? And how did what seemed an adequate protective attitude turn into a problem, with daily crying and a drop in school performance? A comprehensive analysis makes it easier to plan a focused intervention, but one that produces equally comprehensive results in the shortest time possible.

General Aspects of Child Therapy and Final Considerations

With regard to its structuring, starting from what happens in the therapeutic session, the application of FAP in children does not differ significantly from its application in the adult population, as already described above. The difference is in the fact that the goals need to adjust not only to the child's behavior but to what is feasible for him/her according to his/her age and developmental level (Cattivelli et al., 2012), in addition to considering how parents can (and if they can) contribute, both to solving the child's problem and to minimizing the impact that family problems may be having on the child. Another point of consideration is the knowledge of what certain circumstances or adverse conditions usually generate in children. There are situations in which knowledge of certain behavioral patterns, based on scientific evidence, leads the therapist to formulate more appropriate hypotheses and thus better plan his interventions.

The great contribution of FAP lies in the precise description of what therapists should do and how to do it. However, little is still known about the important variables that direct therapeutic decisions, although research is being conducted in this direction (Romero-Porras et al., 2018). What leads a therapist to choose one direction or another within the therapeutic interaction has been a topic of study and discussion for some time now (Moura & Venturelli, 2004). Intervention with children based on FAP principles allows child therapists to apply scientific principles and work consistently within behavior analysis.

In fact, much of what Kohlenberg and Tsai (1991) managed to systematize and conceptualize in relation to clinical practice in behavior therapy has already been used for some time, in another way and under other theoretical bases, by psychotherapists of various approaches. For example, Oaklander (1978), working within the Gestalt approach, describes in his book a psychotherapeutic work with children, based mainly on the experiences that occur during the session and in his relationship with them. His approach could well be considered a practical and very functional way of applying the strategies arising from the FAP in children's clinical practice. Although technically useful, such a work does not have the purpose and, therefore, does not contain the conceptual basis that subsidizes the proposal of Kohlenberg and Tsai (1991). This is the great gain for behavioral therapists, who can increasingly expand and intensify their intervention in a consistent and scientific manner and create stronger links between clinical practice and behavior analysis.

Finally, a word about the therapist. To be ready for this type of work implies the development of his self-knowledge and a constant self-evaluation and support, if possible through personal psychotherapy or therapeutic supervisions. Without this, the analysis of the therapeutic relationship can be something complex, costly, and risky, even in work with children. For this is the proposal of FAP: that the special and unique relationship between client and therapist is the main vehicle for change.

References

Cattivelli, R., Tirelli, V., Berardo, F., & Perini, S. (2012). Promoting appropriate behavior in daily life contexts using functional analytic psychotherapy in early-adolescent children. *International Journal of Behavioral Consultation and Therapy, 7*(2–3), 25–32. https://doi.org/10.1037/h0100933

Conte, F. C. S. (1993). A Terapia Infantil na Clínica Comportamental. In Encontro de Terapeutas Comportamentais de São Paulo: USP (Ed.), *Palestra proferida e não publicada*. Versão ampliada para fins didáticos.

Conte, F. C. S., & Regra, J. A. G. (2000). Psicoterapia comportamental infantil: novos aspectos. In E. F. M. Silvares (Ed.), *Estudos de caso em psicoterapia clínica comportamental infantil* (pp. 79–134). Papirus.

Fernández Parra, A., & Ferro García, R. (2006). La Psicoterapia Analítico-Funcional: una aproximación contextual funcional al tratamiento psicológico. *Edupsykhé, 5*(2), 203–229.

Ferster, C. B. (1979). Psychotherapy from the standpoint of a behaviorist. In J. D. Keehn (Ed.), *Psychopathology in animals: Research and clinical implications*. Academic Press.

Hayes, S. C. (1987). A contextual approach to therapeutic change. In N. S. Jacobson (Ed.), *Psychotherapist in clinical practice: Cognitive and behavioral perspectives* (pp. 327–387). Guilford Press.

Hayes, S. (2004). Acceptance and commitment therapy, relational frame theory, and the third wave of behavioral and cognitive therapies. *Behavior Therapy, 35*, 639–665.

Kohlenberg, R. J., & Tsai, N. (1987). Functional analytic psychotherapy. In N. S. Jacobson (Ed.), *Psychotherapist in clinical practice: Cognitive and behavioral perspectives* (pp. 388–443). Guilford.

Kohlenberg, R. J., & Tsai, M. (1991). Functional analytic psychotherapy: Creating intense and curative therapeutic relationships. *Plenum Press*. https://doi.org/10.1007/978-0-387-70855-3

Moura, C. B., & Conte, F. C. S. (1997). *A psicoterapia analítico-funcional aplicada a terapia comportamental infantil: A participação da criança* (Vol. 4, pp. 131–144). Torre de Babel (UEL).

Moura, C. B., & Venturelli, M. B. (2004). Direcionamentos para a condução do processo terapêutico comportamental com crianças. *Revista Brasileira de Terapia Comportamental e Cognitiva, 6*(1), 17–30. Recuperado em 23 de agosto de 2022, de http://pepsic.bvsalud.org/scielo.php?script=sci_arttext&pid=S1517-55452004000100003&lng=pt&tlng=pt

Oaklander, V. (1978). *Windows to our children: A gestalt approach to children and adolescents*. The Gestalt Journal Press.

Pérez Álvarez, M. (2006). La terapia de conducta de tercera generación. *Edupsykhé, 5*(2), 159–172.

Romero-Porras, J., Obando-Posada, D., Hernández-Barrios, A., & Velasco-Pinzón, D. (2018). Functional analytic psychotherapy among mothers with children with disruptive behavior. *Clínica y Salud, 29*(1), 39–44. https://doi.org/10.5093/clysa2018a7

Chapter 10
Levels of Therapeutic Intervention in Psychotherapy with Children

Cynthia Borges de Moura and Isabel Sá

The literature on child therapy is full of information on procedures and behavioral strategies to be implemented in sessions with children, and the market today also provides many options of playful materials. However, it is necessary to consider that the outcome of the therapy depends on the correct choice of techniques and the therapist's skill in their management (Braga & Vandenberghe, 2006). The skill involves deliberate, purposeful interventions by the therapist – the so-called specific factors, in the sense of managing the child's repertoire to model the desired changes. And this implies, in part, in the interpersonal relationship established between the therapist and his/her small client – nonspecific factors.

In adult therapy, the empirical study of specific factors (intentional actions of the therapist, application of procedures aimed at definite changes), some time ago, began to give way to the so-called nonspecific factors, the inherent characteristics of a constructive human relationship (such as mutual self-disclosure and acceptance), which equally affect the outcome of psychotherapy (Chambless & Ollendick, 2001; Luborsky et al., 2002). But what about in child psychotherapy? How can these factors be integrated, given the differential characteristics of treatment at this stage of development?

This chapter aims to discuss the verbal interventions that take place in an interactional context between the therapist and the child. What does the therapist say, when faced with a given behavior, at an early or intermediate moment of the process? How does he decide which level of intervention to focus on at that moment? The content, how the child solves problems, how he relates to people, or how he is relating to the therapist in the here and now?

C. B. de Moura (✉)
Universidade Estadual do Oeste do Paraná, Foz do Iguaçu, Brazil
e-mail: cynthia.moura@unioeste.br

I. Sá
Universidade de Lisboa, Lisboa, Portugal

Zaro et al. (1980) described four levels of psychotherapeutic interaction, which evolve from the discussion of the content to the discussion of the therapist-client relationship, considering that therapy occurs in a context of interpersonal relationship. In this sense, he notes that the client's behavior affects the therapist's and vice versa and that this can be used to benefit the change process.

Some years later, Kohlenberg and Tsai (1987) presented a systematized proposal from the theoretical and practical point of view in the same direction, the intervention based on the analysis of the therapeutic relationship: functional analytic psychotherapy (FAP). This proposal assumes that "if the client emits the problematic behavior within the context of the therapeutic relationship it is because this one keeps a functional similarity with his daily life environment" (Braga & Vandenberghe, 2006, p. 309). In other words, the problem that brought the client to therapy will appear in the therapeutic relationship and may be worked on live, thus putting the "nonspecific variables" in the foreground.

Exactly 10 years later, Moura and Conte (1997) analyzed how the proposal by Kohlenberg and Tsai could be used in clinical practice with children. But considering that the divisions and definitions of the levels of intervention presented by Zaro et al. (1980) are didactically useful to therapists, mainly to child therapists, this chapter aims at rereading these levels, in the context of psychotherapy with children. Being aware of the levels of therapeutic interaction that can be established makes the therapist better able to assess and decide when and how to respond in more complex ways to their client.

First Level: Content of the Material Brought to the Session by the Client

This is, according to Zaro et al. (1980), the most obvious and "safe" therapeutic material to work with the client. It is a necessary focus for the therapist to evaluate what is happening in the client's life; what he does, thinks, and feels; the context that triggered the problem; and what kind of coping resource he usually adopts.

The content focus allows the therapist to efficiently obtain information about specific behaviors, reactions, context, and consequences produced in the physical and social environment. However, this level of approach is of limited value because if the therapist deals only with the content of what is reported, the therapist's understanding will be restricted to what the client identifies as the problem or to the part of the problem that the client is able to recognize. And this, in the case of children, can be very limiting.

An example is a 10-year-old girl, attending the second grade of elementary school with a complaint of frequent crying at least three times a week, both at home and at school. The therapist asked her to tell about the last time she cried, and the child reported that she fell off her bicycle and cut her foot. According to the girl, her aunt came to see her because she cried a lot and said that "a girl this age does not cry like that" and that it was common to fall off a bicycle. The therapist decided to work on this content and asked: "and what do you think of what your aunt said? Do you agree that a 10-year-old girl does not cry?"

The therapist in the above cut had already understood that the situations evoking crying were minimal annoyances, pain, or embarrassment. Perhaps this is why she chose to work with the content of the aunt's talk to the child, maintaining the same reasoning: that her response was exacerbated for the situation. Several therapists could deal with this child's account in a similar way, and there is nothing wrong with that. Generally, dealing with the content of the client's account is a known, comfortable way and brings access to other important contents. In the above cut, the therapist could perceive that the child "had no idea" of the inadequacy of the frequency and intensity of her emotional responses to common situations in her life.

Zaro et al. (1980) state that the urgency to understand events and how the client coped with them in order to thus provide helpful responses that promote rapid change may increase the likelihood that the therapist will intervene at the content level.

To understand the problem from a different perspective requires more interaction time. As the sessions go on, and the behavioral patterns of your small client are repeated, the therapist will have his or her own impressions of what is happening, what the problem actually is, and may choose to intervene at another level.

Second Level: Customer's Problem-Solving Style

Viewing the client's behavior in therapy as a sample of his behavior in general, outside of this context, requires a more complex kind of analysis. The therapist, in the previous example, might view the report of the episode of the child's "whining after a bicycle tip-over in which she cut her foot" (not actually a cut) as a sample of the larger therapeutic problem.

When the therapist chooses to work at this level, they need to respond not to the content but to how the child resolves the situation and what strategies they employ and their functionality to actually solve the problem. Observe the same interaction in which the therapist gives a different response.

Child: I fell off my bike and cut my foot, I cried a lot!
Therapist: Wow, let me see where you cut it? (Child shows a skinned foot.)
Therapist continues: Well, I think in this case, three things happened: I fell off the bike, I skinned my foot, and I cried a lot. And this last thing doesn't seem to have solved the first two, does it?

See that the therapist subtly reformulates the child's interpretation of the injury, changing "cut by skinning," without confronting the child with the exaggeration of her response. Nor is she disregarding crying as an acceptable response in a bicycle fall situation, she just sets up "outrageous and dramatic crying" (as defined by the mother) as "crying a lot." The option is to focus on the child's repetitive pattern of behavior, highlighting the way he reacts to problems and that does not produce effective results.

In fact, it does! This response generates attention, care, and help from the adult. Probably, these consequences are maintaining the problem, even with the punishments (scolding, punishment) that he receives afterwards. But at this level of approach, the therapist uses one piece of information or one report as a basis for intervening on a larger problem. The exacerbated emotional response is probably a consequence of a deficit in autonomy, problem-solving, and coping repertoires, which she should already have, hence the interpretation of the adults in her social environment as "inappropriate for her age." Another example:

Child: Yesterday at school I couldn't put a puzzle together and I cried. Then the teacher came to give me tips, to help me.
Therapist (in a good mood): Whining strikes again! Oh, dear, how could you get help without turning on the faucet?

In this second example, the therapist confronts the child again with the emission of the problem behavior and requires from him an assertive response that could be emitted in the same situation, which would produce the same consequence and would be more adequate for his developmental level. If the therapist decides to intervene at this level, it is because the alternative and assertive response has already been taught and trained. Otherwise, such intervention, besides being inadequate, would be extremely nontherapeutic!

As the therapist interacts more with the child, he becomes more aware of the problems that should be focused on, as well as of the steps to be taken with the client towards the target responses, that is, the intermediate responses that should be part of the modeling process (Zaro et al., 1980). In this way, alternative and varied problem-solving responses can be taught and their use required both in sessions and in small everyday situations brought by the child.

Third Level: The Client's Interpersonal Relationship Style

The psychotherapeutic context can be seen as a stage to observe how the client relates to other people. Zaro et al. (1980) state that the "therapist-patient" characteristics present in a treatment relationship make it different in many ways from typical interactions between people. Nevertheless, it will be possible to get a very real sample of how your small client deals with interpersonal relationships with other adults and with his peers through the way he interacts with the therapist in session.

Does the child seem to strive to please you or get your approval no matter what the cost? Does he seem to resist all your efforts to help him and your suggestions for behavioral alternatives, with phrases like, "It's no use! No one really understands me"? Does your small client argue with or oppose your proposed activities in an effort to dispute who is in control? Does he/she praise you as a "good friend" and then engage in a long story to justify why he/she won't get what you ask of him/her?

Understanding how your actions affect your client will give the therapist a significant advantage in producing changes in the desired direction.

Drawing on the relational dimension to respond to the client, the therapist could handle the same situation in the following way:

Child: I fell off my bike and cut my toe, I cried a lot!
Therapist: Wow, let me see where you cut it? (Child shows a skinned foot.)
Therapist continues, "I see a splinter foot...Let me ask you something: Do you cry every time a little something goes wrong? Or when someone does or says something you don't like? Is that going to happen here with us? (And adds in a good-humored tone): Oh, oh, oh, don't turn on the crying here!"

There are many ways in which a therapist can use this level of analysis to facilitate treatment. In this case, the therapist hypothesizing that the confrontation she is making could trigger crying tries to block that response with good humor before it happens, thus creating a context for a different, perhaps even incompatible, response. If, for example, the child laughs at the way the therapist said "crying," she can reinforce this response in the sense of confrontation: "That's it! How about we laugh at our problems once in a while? It might work! Shall we try it?"

Intervening at this level is particularly useful for children whose problems revolve around the way they relate socially, both with adults and with other children. As illustrated in the last example, the therapeutic relationship makes it possible to directly or indirectly observe the client's problematic interpersonal style, signaling an alternative in the opposite direction, which can be trained in the moment, in the heat (or freshness!) of the situation.

Zaro et al. (1980) state that the advantage of intervening at this level is that it enables the therapist to correct "blind spots" concerning the way in which the client affects other people. For example:

Child: Yesterday at school I couldn't put a puzzle together and I cried. Then the teacher came to give me tips, to help me.
Therapist: I'm going to tell you something kind of boring, but important. When someone cries in front of us, it usually sensitizes us to help. But when the person *always* cries, others get bored...and move away...soon the person will be without help and without friends too! Have you ever thought about that?

The therapist above already risks showing the child how others are likely to perceive her and what the consequences of this behavior will be in the medium term. The intention is that this information will affect the child's behavior in the desired direction. Importantly, the therapist warns that her intervention will not be pleasant. This is a tactic that facilitates the acceptance of the confrontation, because the therapist shows that she cares and it is her role to point out the "boring parts," so that change can occur. The approach is complex, and there is rarely a clear right or wrong way to work at this level. The therapist may become aware of a pattern in the client's interpersonal response, but may be unsure how to address it or what would be a productive time to do so. If this is the case, wait one more session, and when you do venture out, use the "laying the groundwork" tactic illustrated in the example.

Fourth Level: How the Client's Behavior Affects the Therapist

Viewing psychotherapy as an interaction between people assumes that just as your behavior affects the client's behavior, the client's behavior also affects you. Recognizing your personal reactions to the client's behavior and using them to achieve therapy goals adds a fourth level of therapeutic intervention.

Vandenberghe (2017, p. 221) states that "strategic disclosure of the feelings the client evokes in the therapist may be a productive option, but one must consider how these feelings resemble or are distinct from the feelings of other people in the client's life and how disclosure may impact the client."

Imagine how it feels to be a therapist interacting with a 10-year-old who cries at every little difficulty? It is quite possible that after an initial empathic reaction, the therapist may begin to feel frustrated or upset. In that case, he may externalize a personal reaction to the client for the purpose of helping him become more aware of how his behavior affects him as well as other people. For example:

Child: Yesterday, at school, I couldn't put a puzzle together and I cried. Then the teacher came to give me tips, to help me.
Therapist: Oh no! Again? We've already talked and rehearsed together what to do in these situations! Why didn't you ask for help? I'm sure your teacher would come to your aid if you asked her in words.

The evaluation of his own emotional reaction may be the starting point for the therapist to formulate a response to the client. In the cut above, understanding that the "inassertive crying" is related to the lack of coping repertoire, and admitting that this behavior frustrates and annoys him in the same way as the teacher or mother, the therapist decides to react to the child's resistance to implement the new strategies exhaustively rehearsed.

Vandenberghe (2017) cautions therapists to be careful and check what aspects of the client's behavior they are responding to. If the immediate impact of this interaction on the client is likely to result in an increased frequency of healthier behavior in the client's daily life, then it is worth taking a chance on this level of intervention. If, on the other hand, the therapist identifies that their reaction has more to do with their difficulty in dealing with "whiny children" who are resistant to change or that this child's behavior irritates them because they seem lazy and manipulative, it is better not to respond to it. It would not be therapeutic to support intervention on such feelings.

The therapist must ask himself whether his reactions to the client's behavior in question are relevant to the goals of therapy. This is the determining factor in deciding how and when to use his personal feelings as an intervention strategy. As long as he has recognized his feelings as legitimate to the interaction, he can use them to analyze and intervene at the level of the therapeutic relationship.

In the same example, still within the intervention at this level, the therapist should also consider what else might have generated this feeling besides the child's resistance. This can lead to the recognition that he may have focused the therapy on training alternative responses without considering the variables that control his small client's response in the natural environment. In that case, he might choose a different verbalization. For example:

Child: Yesterday at school I couldn't put a puzzle together and I cried. Then the teacher came to give me tips, to help me.
Therapist: Wow. I keep asking myself why is it that with me you can say what you want without crying, but not at school? What is it that happens there that we haven't found out yet?

When realizing that his frustration may be the result of a "technical failure in the process" and that the child is trying to correspond to the therapist's expectations, but is not succeeding due to other variables not considered, the therapist may take a step back and analyze this together with his client. Many times their feelings will give them clues about their own behavior as therapist, which will need to be modified for the benefit of the client, as in the above cut.

According to Kohlenberg and Tsai (1987), just as the client introduces his own characteristic style and personal problems into the therapeutic relationship, so does the therapist. For this reason, the use of this level of analysis is recommended only after careful consideration. Although few therapists make the mistake of imprudently attributing their own idiosyncratic responses to their clients, many sin by going in the opposite direction, establishing a distant and impersonal relationship. With children, besides being unproductive, this is also disastrous.

When the child begins to abandon his inadequate behavior patterns and to develop more appropriate interaction alternatives, that is the moment for the therapist to value such progress and feel reinforced by it (Moura & Conte, 1997). In this sense, a hypothetical response that would contemplate this aspect could be:

Child: Yesterday at school I was able to hold...I raised my hand and asked if the teacher could repeat the explanation.
Therapist: Wow...I'm the one who's going to cry now! With emotion! What's up?
Child: Then she said yes, and other children said they didn't understand either. She explained again and I understood.
Therapist: Finally the score is reversing! You 1 vs. Crying 0!

Being able to naturally reinforce the client's improvements by feeling reinforced by them is an important therapeutic skill according to Kohlenberg and Tsai (1987), as it increases the likelihood that the therapist will use his or her personal resources in a more conscious and therapeutic way, always bearing in mind that a reinforcing relationship between client and therapist is fundamental to the process.

Much of what Kohlenberg and Tsai (1987, 1991) systematized in relation to clinical practice in behavior therapy has already been used for some time by other psychotherapists (Zaro et al., 1980) and professionals from other theoretical bases (Oaklander, 1978). The last author describes, from a gestalt approach, how to develop a psychotherapeutic work with children, based mainly on the experiences during the session and its relationship with the child.

The levels of intervention exposed, as well as the examples presented, serve didactic functions. In practice, they may even occur more or less in this order, because they depend on a more frequent contact with the child and the establishment of intimacy in the relationship, but they do not constitute stages. The aim was to illustrate to the child therapist how to approach the report, the behavior, and the therapeutic process of children at different levels, so that the relationship with their young clients may produce the learning of productive repertoires for both.

References

Braga, G. L. B., & Vandenberghe, L. (2006). Abrangência e função da relação terapêutica na terapia comportamental. *Estudos de Psicologia, 23*(3), 307–314.
Chambless, D. L., & Ollendick, T. H. (2001). Empirically supported psychological interventions: Controversies and evidence. *Annual Review of Psychology, 52*(1), 685–716.
Kohlenberg, R. J., & Tsai, N. (1987). Functional analytic psychotherapy. In N. S. Jacobson (Ed.), *Psychotherapist in clinical practice: Cognitive and behavioral perspectives*. Guilford.
Kohlenberg, R. J., & Tsai, M. (1991). Functional analytic psychotherapy: Creating intense and curative therapeutic relationships. *Plenum Press*. https://doi.org/10.1007/978-0-387-70855-3
Luborsky, L., Rosenthal, R., Diguer, L., Andrusyna, T. P., Berman, J. S., Levitt, J. T., Seligman, D. A., & Krausse, E. D. (2002). The dodo bird verdict is alive and well - mostly. Clinical psychology. *Science and Practice, 9*(1), 2–12.
Moura, C. B., & Conte, F. C. S. (1997). A psicoterapia analítico-funcional aplicada à terapia comportamental infantil: A participação da criança. *Torre de Babel., 4*(1), 131–144.
Oaklander, V. (1978). *Windows to our children: A gestalt approach to children and adolescents*. The Gestalt Journal Press.
Vandenberghe, L. (2017). Três faces da Psicoterapia Analítica Funcional: Uma ponte entre análise do comportamento e terceira onda. *Revista Brasileira de Terapia Comportamental e Cognitiva, 19*(3), 206–2019.
Zaro, J. S., Barach, R., Nedelman, D. J., & Dreiblat, I. S. (1980). *Introdução à prática psicoterapêutica*. (Trad. Lucio Roberto Marzagão). Edusp.

Chapter 11
Contact with Schools: Objectives, Limits, and Care

Ligia Lacava Barros and Carolina Toledo Piza

According to Regra (2000), the children's clinic is a therapeutic process that covers more than one client: besides the child, it also involves his/her parents. However, a basic aspect of behavior analysis is the understanding of the individual's behaviors as a product of interaction with the environment (Todorov, 2007). Thus, when it comes to children, the concept of environment is expanded and extended to the school context, as an important environment where they spend much of the day. Therefore, the goal of the child behavioral clinic also includes changing the child's behavioral relationships and reinforcement contingencies within the school environment in order to enable the client's social and academic aspects.

Considering this important partnership, the therapist's contact with schools is essential, even when the referral for care has arisen from a need by parents or other professionals/specialists who have evaluated and/or are also monitoring the child. For example, a child with oral language alteration may already be assisted by a specialist who works in this area (in Brazil, they are usually speech therapists), and another child with school issues may have the complementary monitoring of a psycho-pedagogist or school psychologist. In this way, when we begin our work, it is a fundamental part of the process to establish contact with the network of professionals who accompany the client, in order to understand the reason for referral, how they have acted, and what the scope of their therapeutic planning is (Hunter & Dunders, 2007). If the therapeutic work was a referral from the school, it is worth knowing all the elements that will be important for the behavioral clinic identified by the school.

As this chapter focuses on exploring the aims, limits, and care of school contact, we will focus more on this important participant in the child's network. Contact

L. L. Barros (✉)
Universidade Federal de São Paulo, São Paulo, Brazil

C. T. Piza
Private Practice, São Paulo, Brazil

with the school has two main objectives. The first is to raise important elements for the functional analysis. As school is one of the main learning and socialization environments for children, it is a space in which they develop behaviors related to organization, responsibility, and academic skills. Thus, the data brought by school professionals are essential to broaden the understanding of our client's functioning. Through this contact, we seek to identify his behavioral components and understand how relationships are established between the child and his peers, as well as behaviors involving learning processes and study habits. We aim to investigate how, when, and if the teaching process occurs, in its various contingencies (Prado et al., 2012). Understanding the child's attitude in the classroom and outside it, respect for rules and peers, involvement in academic activities, the concentration time required and performed by the child in various activities, and his/her attitude when facing challenging and improvised situations are some of the important behaviors that help the therapist to establish a functional analysis (Sidman, 2006).

The second objective is more related to networking, which aims to strengthen the partnership between school-therapist-client-family (and the other possible professionals that make up the network). Studies for over a decade have reinforced positive effects on student development and learning when this family-school network is integrated (Smith et al., 2020). The partnership improves academic performance as well as social, emotional, and behavioral experiences (Sheridan & Gutkin, 2000). Expanding this network to include the therapist as part of that partnership makes this process even more supportive. In many cases, complaints may refer to lack of commitment, difficulties in the academic sphere, or inappropriate behaviors in the school environment, which, to be managed, necessarily need support and exposure to this environment. For example, if we consider the case of a student who presents academic difficulties, or even a confirmed diagnosis of dyslexia, depending on the complaint and the complexity of the picture, it is necessary to co-construct, with the various participants in the network, possible adaptations or support that will allow this student to be better accommodated to the school environment. It is necessary that this decision is also shared with the client and his family, so that it can then be discussed and adapted by the school. We can also consider a second scenario, in which the client has difficulty socializing with his peers. In this case, again, it is important that the network partnership is well established, to consider how much the school can contribute (either with more direct interventions or observations from a distance) to expand the positive models of interaction that will be offered to the child and his peers.

The initial contact with the school team can be made at different times. In certain contexts, it is suggested that it occurs at the very beginning of the therapeutic process, concomitant with the initial sessions with the family and child, always after their consent. This usually occurs when the child has been referred at the school's request, so contact is usually established in the first weeks of care, even if there is not yet a fully formulated therapeutic plan. In these cases, the visit aims to establish an initial relationship, in which we listen to the school staff (much more than taking ready-made guidelines), to understand their pedagogical proposal, as well as their view on the student: the main complaints and description of behaviors (desirable and undesirable) presented in that environment. Only after this meeting, we began to formulate a plan that also includes goals for the school context (Meltzer, 2010).

In other cases, when the central complaint is not directly related to the school environment, contact with the school may be made some time after the initial sessions with the parents and child. In this case, the therapist already has relevant data and can combine them with the aspects brought by the school or add new behaviors presented by the client to his planning, considering the different environments and variables. It is very common for the child to present undesirable behaviors in the family environment but not at school. For example, parents may complain that the child is very aggressive and defiant when at home, but in some cases, this behavior is not evidenced at school. The opposite may also occur – although it is less frequent – of parents claiming that the child presents behaviors at school that they do not observe in everyday situations.

Let us illustrate with the case of Mary, a 9-year-old girl whose family sought therapy because the school claimed that the child was withdrawn and not very participatory in group activities (with her classmates) and vehemently avoided situations of highlighting and exposure during classes when the teacher requested her participation. According to the parents, Mary was an extremely communicative and outgoing girl, and her attitudes did not match the complaints, although they noticed more restlessness and tension during homework assignments. In this case, it was important to strengthen the relationship with the school to understand the reason for such behaviors and subsequently explain to the parents the contingencies that led Mary to react in such a way.

As already mentioned, when the therapist makes the first (or any) contact with the school, it is essential that the parents are in agreement and have consented, as they are the clients and responsible for the child. In general, they usually understand the importance of this approach with the school; however, there are some exceptions, in which families resist the contact. In these cases, it is important to respect the family's opinion and gradually justify it, reinforcing the importance of the link with the school for the best progress of the case.

When parents consent to this communication, in most cases, the ideal is to seek the educational guidance team, or school psychologist, which monitors aspects related to the psychosocial development of students. Some schools do not have this team in their structure to meet the demands, and, in this case, the contact is made directly with the educational manager or with the school board. When we are working with children attending Elementary I, whenever possible, it is also interesting to request the participation of the class teacher. In some cases, the school has a support department for inclusive students, and contact can also be made with other professionals (specialists) who are part of this therapeutic network.

Contact with the school should be made, however, in a very cautious manner, aiming at the confidential aspects of both parties. As mentioned, the clinician needs to remember that his clients are the child and his parents and that aspects revealed to the school may harm the family. Thus, in some cases, it is also necessary to have the family's permission to share personal information of family functioning, and, if denied, the therapist must consent to this choice. In these cases, the focus should be on behaviors related to the learning environment.

Similarly, relevant information brought by the school should be passed on to parents only with the consent of the school professionals and with care not to expose third parties, such as teachers, coordinators, and the like. It is also worth reinforcing that, according to the association's code of ethics, any report prepared by the clinician, which contains information regarding the child and his/her family, can only be sent to the school with the family's consent. Therefore, it is essential that the parents read and authorize the sharing of the document before it is sent. If they choose not to share certain information, the clinician can make a brief report version to deliver to the school and a second, more extensive version to share with specialists and doctors who may eventually follow up on the case. It is also suggested that the clinician be careful not to disclose information contained in the reports prepared by him or herself or by other professionals who evaluated the client, in case this sharing has been denied by the family members.

The frequency with which you will contact the school varies from case to case. It is important to note that, even if the child does not present issues related to academic performance or undesirable behaviors at school, it is important to maintain telephone contact from time to time, coupled with a few face-to-face meetings per year.

However, in cases where the school is directly related to the complaint, contact with it should happen more frequently, since part of the therapeutic goals involves this physical and social environment. Take case 2, for example: Nate is referred to therapy at the school's request, with parental consent. The school reports that the client has been exhibiting separation anxiety disorder, not being able to attend school every day of the week nor during the entire school term.

In this case, the clinician will need to establish frequent contact with the school to develop systematic exposures that enable Nate's return to the school environment, relying on family participation when necessary. In this scenario, it may be necessary to observe the child's interaction in his school environment. To assist in this process, before making the observation in loco, the school may be provided with a behavior assessment tool that will help guide which behaviors will be analyzed during the visit. There are a number of behavior observation scales, and some even have more than one version for the people accompanying the client.

For example, this is the case of the SNAP-IV scale (Matos et al., 2006), aimed at investigating signs and symptoms of ADHD, which has one version to be completed by the client and another for parents and/or school staff (teachers and coordinators). Another suggestion is the SDQ (Strengths and Difficulties Questionnaire), which assesses the behavioral characteristics of children and adolescents, as well as the presence of symptoms leading to the diagnosis of psychiatric disorders (Saur, 2012).

It is essential for therapists to be clear about which signs and symptoms they want to explore, in order to define the best scale to be used, which they can fill in themselves during their visit to the school. In situations where the therapist needs to investigate very specific aspects, the therapist can prepare his/her own questionnaire (which will be more qualitative in nature), listing the aspects he/she intends to understand via the school. You can also formulate an observation script with the behaviors you wish to observe during your visit and record how often the client emits them. In this case, one way would be to list behaviors expected by the child in the school environment, such as "relates to peers," "is asked by others," and "responds to verbal requests," evaluating whether "he emits these behaviors with or without intervention," "how often," etc.

Let us analyze another example, which will be called case 3: Joseph is referred to therapy by his parents for presenting behavioral issues in the family environment. He is described as an aggressive child who confronts his parents, fights a lot with his younger brother, and eventually has "tantrums" when he is contradicted. When contacting the school, the report is that the client does not present disruptive behaviors, respects rules imposed without questioning, delivers the activities on time, and has a good relationship with peers and teachers and coordination.

According to the brief report, it can be noted that, in all the cases illustrated above, contact with the school is necessary; however, in the third case, the focus of monitoring differs from the first two, in which the school environment presents aversive contingencies that trigger inappropriate behavior. Thus, in this last example, contact with another environment (other than the family) helps to confirm that the child has more adaptive repertoires, which reinforces the need to guide the family, offering as models chains of contingencies similar to those of the school. Contact with the school, in this case, despite being an important part of the partnership, does not need to occur in the same frequency as in the previous examples, because the priority interventions should take place in the family environment. In cases 1 and 2, however, the analyst aims to observe (in loco) and understand why the stimuli presented in the school environment evoke poorly adaptive behavior as a consequence. In these scenarios, therapist-school contact should occur more frequently and systematically, to observe not only what the student does but also the relationships between his behavior, the aspects that precede it, and those that arise as a consequence of the environment, promoting his learning, both in the physical and social spheres (Prado et al., 2012).

Let's reflect back on the first case, considering that Mary has exhibited avoidance behaviors during situations of greater exposure in the classroom. After some time of follow-up, the therapist began to observe that such behaviors were the consequence of a significant school deficit, especially in activities involving reading and writing. Thus, she referred the child to a complementary neuropsychological multidisciplinary evaluation, which further investigated the child's cognitive and behavioral profile, focusing on learning processes. The evaluation data confirmed a specific reading learning disorder, also known as dyslexia, pointing to a significant deficit in reading and writing skills (alteration in reading fluency and comprehension, phonological and orthographic changes – when reading and writing), in operational memory tasks (requiring mental manipulation), and those involving greater phonological processing and rapid *automatic* naming (RAN tasks), with a slow response to intervention when compared to the client's level of intelligence and schooling (Cruz-Rodrigues, et al., 2014; Shaywitz & Shaywitz, 2005; American Psychiatric Association, 2013; Piza et al., 2009).

Given this diagnostic confirmation, the behavior analyst can act as case manager and resume meetings with the school coordinator, reinforcing the areas of greater cognitive and behavioral weakness confirmed by the evaluation, and then establish new therapeutic goals (together with the coordinator), aiming to expand the educators' knowledge and conduct about the case (Hunter & Dunders, 2007). When a solid partnership is established between therapist and school, it is possible to collaboratively build strategies that will reduce aversive behaviors while promoting the expansion, consolidation, and refinement of new behaviors acquired and more appropriate to the student.

In this particular example, it is known that psychoeducation is a fundamental stage of the process, since students with learning disorders can often be misunderstood and misinterpreted by parents and school staff, because they usually show notorious discrepancy in expressing and understanding information orally, when compared to the quality of their production and written language. In addition, students with school difficulties (whether or not they have a confirmed diagnosis) often adopt behaviors of indifference, avoidance, and evasion (being seen as "lazy" or "sloppy") or even arrogance in the face of "not knowing."

Thus, understanding the functioning profile of these individuals helps the network of parents-specialists-school to design specific and more appropriate strategies for the client, allowing more appropriate and less aversive contingencies to be modeled that access the client's true knowledge and potential. For example, again considering case 1 (Mary), after diagnostic confirmation, the behavior analyst met again with the specialists (in this case, the neuropsychologist), parents, and client to present the proposals for adaptation that she would like to suggest to the school team. Based on the multidisciplinary assessment, it was observed that the student would benefit from facilitating strategies for reading and textual comprehension, for example, the use of rubrics or summaries (prompts) with guiding questions and steps for problem-solving (plan, organize, and self-monitor production); bold keywords in texts/sentences to hold her attention; the study through short activities, with repetition of content; and audiovisual support (when possible) to assist the absorption of content and quality of performance. It was also considered the reduction of more complex/longer statements, fractioned into smaller parts to help her reflect on the content, stimulating abilities to plan her action before executing it. Another suggestion was that Mary should take tests in quieter environments and have ample time, allowing breaks when a drop in performance or increase in anxiety was observed.

Upon exposing such guidelines to the client and her parents, Mary reported that she would not like to take all the tests in another setting. In this case, the therapist realized that such a strategy would increase her aversion to the assessment context (where the client felt "very different from her peers"). In this case, therapist and client agreed with the school that she would only take some of the tests (concerning the subjects in which she had more difficulty) outside the classroom. This example demonstrates that it is essential for the behavior analyst to know his client and be able to identify the contingencies that increase or decrease a behavior so that strategies and interventions are carefully chosen, avoiding "ready-made" orientations that prioritize the diagnosis and not the client's profile (Barkley, 2012).

Furthermore, it is important that the behavior analyst also deepens his/her knowledge of the most frequent neurodevelopmental disorders so that, when necessary, he/she can also suggest adaptations and accessibility focused on teaching technologies (Hunter and Dunders, 2007). Integrating their knowledge about the client's behavioral profile with specific characteristics of these childhood conditions will allow professionals to offer more realistic, personalized, and fundamental strategies to expand and adapt teaching methods that may include complementary resources, such as audiovisual proposals and computer tools (Prado et al., 2012).

Finally, it is worth noting that when reflecting on school guidelines, it is essential to consider the school's profile, as well as its openness and flexibility in accepting external suggestions. In Marina's case in particular, the specialists had established a good link with the school team, so they knew that such adaptations would be possible and well accepted. However, there are situations where, unfortunately, the school staff are less willing to discuss suggestions proposed by specialists. In these cases, it is important to respect this space, but clearly expose the student's needs, as well as the contingencies that increase his/her inappropriate behaviors. Special care should be taken not to wear out the relationship between the family/student and the school, aiming to strengthen the bond of this network. However, it is also the role of the behavior analyst to consider, realistically, how well the school is prepared to receive and work with the student's needs.

In short, working with children and adolescents requires establishing a bridge with the school and family, as these are the most important environments of socialization for the child. In addition, numerous studies and case reports have confirmed that the success of clinical evolution is very much related to good partnership work, even when the initial complaint did not come from the school.

References

American Psychiatric Association. (2013). *Diagnostic and statistical manual of mental disorders* (5th ed.). https://doi.org/10.1176/appi.books.9780890425596
Barkley, R. A. (2012). *Executive functions: What they are, how they work, and why they evolved.* The Guilford Press.
Cruz-Rodrigues, C., Barbosa, T., Toledo-Piza, C. M. J., Miranda, M. C., & Bueno, O. F. A. (2014). Neuropsychological characteristics of dyslexic children. *Psicologia: Reflexão e Crítica, 27*(3), 539–546.
Hunter, S. J., & Donders, J. (2007). *Pediatric neuropsychological intervention.* Cambridge University Press.
Mattos, P., Serra-Pinheiro, M. A., Rohde, L. A., & Pinto, D. (2006). Apresentação de uma versão em português para uso no Brasil do instrumento MTA-SNAP-IV de avaliação de sintomas de transtorno do déficit de atenção/hiperatividade e sintomas de transtorno desafiador e de oposição. *Revista de Psiquiatria do Rio Grande do Sul, 28*(3), 290–297.
Meltzer, L. (2010). *Promoting executive function in the classroom.* Guilford Press.

Prado, P. S. T., Beffa, M. J., & Gonsales, T. P. (2012). Análise de contingências em situação pedagógica. In J. S. Carmo & M. J. F. X. Ribeiro (Eds.), *Contribuições da análise do comportamento à prática educacional* (1st ed., pp. 87–110). ESETec Editores Associados.

Piza, C. M. J. T., Bueno, O. F. A., & Macedo, E. C. (2009). Perspectivas atuais acerca da dislexia do desenvolvimento: da avaliação ao diagnóstico. In J. M. Montiel & F. C. Capovilla (Eds.), *Atualização em Transtornos de Aprendizagem* (1st ed., pp. 153–166). Artes Médicas.

Regra, J. (2000). Formas de trabalho na psicoterapia infantil: Mudanças ocorridas e novas direções. *Revista Brasileira de Terapia Comportamental e Cognitiva, 2*(1), 79–101.

Saur, A. M., & Loureiro, S. R. (2012). Qualidades psicométricas do Questionário de Capacidades e Dificuldades: revisão da literatura. *Estudos de Psicologia, 29*(4), 619–629.

Shaywitz, S. E. & Shaywitz, B. A. (2005). Dyslexia (Specific Reading Disability). *Biological Psychiatry, 57*, 1301–1309.

Sheridan, S. M., & Gutkin, T. B. (2000). The ecology of school psychology: Examining and changing our paradigm for the 21st century. *School Psychology Review, 29*, 485–502.

Sidman, M. (2006). Fred S. Keller, um reforçador condicionado generalizado. *Revista Brasileira de Análise do Comportamento, 2*, 277–285.

Smith, T. E., Holmes, S. R., Sheridan, S. M., Cooper, J. M., Bloomfield, B. S., & Preast, J. L. (2020). The effects of consultation-based family-school engagement on student and parent outcomes: A meta-analysis. *Journal of Educational and Psychological Consultation*. https://doi.org/10.1080/10474412.2020.1749062

Todorov, J. C. (2007). A Psicologia como o estudo de interações. *Psicologia: Teoria e Pesquisa, 23*(spe), 57–61.

Chapter 12
Interdisciplinary Work in the Care of Children

Liane Jorge de Souza Dahás and Tiffany Moukbel Chaim Avancini

Childhood as a Period of Neurodevelopment: The Importance of a Broad Approach Adapted to the Stages of Life

The period of childhood is marked by major transformations that encompass the affective, social, cognitive, and physical development. Such skills will provide the child's self-sufficiency and the formation of healthy bonds, as well as be part of the development of personality, learning skills, problem-solving skills, and the formulation of new concepts and ideas (Schore & Schore, 2008; Shonkoff & Phillips, 2000).

During childhood and adolescence, the processes of brain development and maturation occur through the selective strengthening or weakening of brain networks. Over time, new neural circuits are being established, and others are being dismantled, undergoing what we call neural pruning. These changes, made possible by brain plasticity, which is nothing more than the brain's ability to modify its connections or reconnect, will lead to the refinement and specialization of brain circuits (Battista et al., 2018). The whole learning processes of the child, including the different experiences to which he/she was exposed and the way physical-cognitive and emotional stimulation was performed, are stimuli that will influence brain plasticity and neurodevelopment. (Nowakowsk & Hayes, 2012; Palkhivala, 2010). Thus, when assessing the child, one should always take into account his/her life history and, at each stage of life, have a different expectation towards his/her emotional and physical behavior since some skills will only be developed at a later stage of development.

L. J. de Souza Dahás (✉)
Paradigma, Center for Behavioral Sciences and Technology, São Paulo, Brazil

T. M. C. Avancini
Private Practice, São Paulo, Brazil

As an example of the peculiarities of each age, we can cite the ability to remain attentive to activities. The expected parameters for this skill vary according to age. In general, up to 6 years old, it is normal for children to have a very short focus time, with numerous interruptions in their activities and the need for an adult to organize the task to be performed. As she gets older, this capacity increases until she is able to stay focused for more than 30 minutes on an activity that, at first, is not very motivating, such as studying (Hood, 1995; Johnson, 1990). If such differences are not taken into account, it is very likely that a misdiagnosis of attention deficit hyperactivity disorder (ADHD) will be attributed to a child with an age-appropriate attentional performance. Studies have shown that younger children within the same school grade, such as those born in December compared to those born in January of the same year, tend to be diagnosed with ADHD in larger numbers, which can lead to misdiagnosis and possible drug treatment of children who would not be indicated for it (Morrow et al., 2012).

Taking into account the complexity of child development, a comprehensive approach to the phenomena of this moment is necessary to take into account all the processes and peculiarities of each phase, supported by the various areas of knowledge (Martins Filho & Martins, 2012). Only in this way, the professional will be able to track possible warning signs and assess the child's evolutionary adequacy, considering all neurodevelopmental and socioemotional development processes.

It is worth noting that transiting through these fields is quite different from having specific knowledge of all areas related to mental health. Once the professional already has in mind all the important aspects to be assessed in the first contacts with the patient (including those that are not present in the initial assessment but that may arise throughout follow-up) and understands the concept of interdisciplinary work, he or she will be able to identify the context in which referral is necessary and will know how to perform adequate teamwork. Knowledge about the functioning of an interdisciplinary team is therefore necessary, as discussed below.

Multi- and Interdisciplinary Teams: Concepts and Practical Developments

The behavior-analytic therapist usually works with teams of several professionals (e.g., treatment of eating disorders in partnership with nutritionists and psychiatrists). In the children's clinic, this practice is also common and highly recommended, taking into account that children are at the beginning of their developmental process, with highly flexible neuronal and motor functioning, as well as behavioral patterns (Papalia et al., 2009).

Within the health sciences, several terms are used to refer to the joint work of professionals coming from different areas. The concepts of multidisciplinarity and interdisciplinarity are described below, and, at the end of this section, it will be explained why the latter term was chosen by the authors as the most appropriate in child mental health care.

Multidisciplinarity is a term used to refer to the set of disciplines studied in parallel, i.e., each professional contributes with their knowledge to the case in question from the knowledge of their discipline of origin (Choi & Pak, 2006). Metaphorically, we can imagine a patchwork quilt, whose composition contains a little piece of cloth from each professional. This is a very common approach in outpatient settings, in which each specialist contributes what is his or her role, without a common formulation of the case among them. The analyses are added up, one by one, and there is usually a leader (usually a physician) who brings them together and decides which should be the priorities and the course of treatment, thus influencing the practice of the other professionals.

For example, in a case of autistic spectrum disorder (ASD), a team composed of a nutritionist, psychiatrist, psychologist, and speech and hearing therapist would be led by the psychiatrist, and, at his discretion, the treatment of food selectivity (nutritionist), language learning (speech and hearing therapist), and basic social skills (psychologist) would be carried out. Numerous opposing perceptions about the case are possible and no synthesis is made. Going back to the example given, the speech-language pathologist may advocate teaching parents not to respond to gesture commands to increase the emission of verbal commands, while the behavior analyst psychologist would certainly advocate first teaching the gesture command and then move on to the vocal command. In this case, the decision of where to start would be of the team leader, based on their own knowledge of the disciplines discussed, since there is no joint case formulation.

Interdisciplinarity relies on disciplines studied in a correlated way, i.e., each professional will bring their experience and theoretical knowledge so that a unique formulation of the case is elaborated (Choi & Pak, 2006). In this team model, there is no leader: all professionals are responsible for the progress of the case and discuss the treatment courses in a linear and nonhierarchical way.

Going back to the example of the child with ASD: the behavior-analytic psychologist could explain to the team the importance of nonvocal command behavior as a precursor to vocal command behavior, as well as echoing. If the team works in an interdisciplinary fashion, there will be a discussion about the importance of simple behaviors being taught before more complex ones in scientific but simpler than behavior-analytic language so that everyone understands. Once the whole team agrees with the premise, the phonoaudiologist may then suggest learning to echo sounds, eventually even touch verbally so that when the nonvocal command is well established, the vocal is inserted into the repertoire.

It is noted that the effects on the course of treatment of multi- and interdisciplinary approaches are quite diverse: in one, dialectical interpretations are possible, and there is a choice by one of the professionals about which would be the most appropriate treatment. In another, the need to formulate a case and make decisions together forces professionals to elaborate a synthetic formulation from among the different interpretations.

The authors of this chapter defend the line that prioritizes the interdisciplinary approach in children's clinical practice. In this approach, each professional can bring specific knowledge of his/her area, which, based on team discussions with all professionals equally involved in the case, will be aligned, adapted, and associated with the patient's demand. This procedure tends to generate greater effectiveness in the individual work of each professional, since it will be performed synergistically with the others, seeking the same objectives.

Interdisciplinary Teams in the Management of Child Psychiatric Disorders

Depending on the symptoms and their functions found in the initial assessment, usually performed by the psychiatrist or therapist, other health professionals may be invited to join the interdisciplinary team, enabling a more specific investigation of issues that relate to the problem presented, but are beyond the scope of psychiatric and psychological intervention.

There are no rules to compose the team of professionals that will treat each condition, and each case must be analyzed individually. However, some psychiatric disorders or neurological conditions require teamwork, with an interdisciplinary approach. Such professionals will be important not only in the treatment but also for the previous process, which involves diagnosis, care with differential diagnoses and possible comorbidities, and therapeutic planning. As an example, we can cite some disorders.

Neurodevelopmental Disorders

Autistic Spectrum Disorder

Autism spectrum disorder (ASD) is characterized by persistent deficits in communication and social interaction in multiple contexts, including deficits in social reciprocity, nonverbal communication behaviors used for social interaction, and skills in developing, maintaining, and understanding relationships. Associated with the impairments in social interaction, for the diagnosis of ASD to be established, there must be the presence of a pattern of restricted and repetitive behaviors, interests, or activities (American Psychiatric Association, 2013).

Considering all the damages that the condition causes, it is easy to identify the need for multiple professionals to carry out an adequate treatment. Thus, among the treatments indicated are psychotherapy with the practice of behavioral interventions and parental guidance, speech therapy focused on speech and language, occupational therapy, and work with sensory integration, monitoring with a child and adolescent psychiatrist and/or neuropediatrician.

There is no specific medication for the treatment of ASD, but several medications can be used to treat symptoms that may accompany the condition, such as excessive irritability and sleep disorders, as well as to address comorbidities, such as anxiety disorders, depressive disorder, and ADHD, among others. When necessary, medication helps to improve the patient's well-being and, thus, brings better conditions for him to respond to the implemented treatments.

Attention Deficit Hyperactivity Disorder

ADHD is a neurodevelopmental disorder defined by a persistent pattern of inattention and/or hyperactivity-impulsivity that generates impairment in functioning and development of the individual. Inattention and disorganization imply inability to stay on task, in addition to appearing not to hear what is being said and missing objects at levels that are inconsistent with age or developmental level. Hyperactivity-impulsivity implies excessive restlessness, restlessness, inability to remain seated, interruption in other people's activities, and inability to wait symptoms that are excessive for age or developmental level (American Psychiatric Association, 2013).

The therapeutic plan for ADHD patients should consider the condition as chronic and may consist essentially of psychopharmacological treatment, performed by a child and adolescent psychiatrist or child neurologist, and behavioral therapy. The therapeutic proposal should always take into account the treatments previously performed, the patient's and family's preferences and concerns, the degree of damage the condition causes, and the patient's current demands. Thus, it is important that the physician and therapist who follow the case perform psychoeducation with the parents and the child and that the existing therapeutic options be clarified.

Still, in many cases, other interventions are also necessary, such as parental training so that parents can help their child to manage the condition and improve their quality of life; the admission of a therapeutic companion or a psychopedagogue to help the child with difficulties secondary to the condition (such as not knowing how to organize, prioritize tasks, learn to study, or even to resume concepts that were lost during the learning process); and a psychomotor or occupational therapist, if the child presents significant impairment in fine and/or gross motor coordination, symptoms commonly associated with the diagnosis.

It is also worth remembering that the presence of comorbidities that may aggravate the condition should always be investigated. Thus, if other contributing causes for inattention are suspected, an evaluation by an audiologist and a central auditory processing test may provide important information for treatment and therapeutic approach.

Specific Learning Disability

This condition is diagnosed when there are specific deficits in an individual's ability to perceive or process information efficiently and accurately. This neurodevelopmental disorder first appears during the formal school years and is characterized by persistent difficulties in learning fundamental academic skills in reading, writing, and/or mathematics, leading to permanent impairment. In general, the individual performance in academic skills is well below the average for his/her age, or acceptable performance levels are achieved only with an immense effort. This condition may also occur in individuals identified as intellectually gifted and will manifest only when learning demands or assessment procedures (e.g., timed tests) present barriers that cannot be overcome by their innate intelligence or compensatory strategies.

For all individuals, specific learning disability can produce lifelong impairments in skill-dependent activities, including occupational performance (American Psychiatric Association, 2013). Diagnosis is based on a synthesis of the child's medical, educational, and family developmental history and history of the learning disability, including past and current manifestations; the impact of the difficulty on academic, occupational, or social functioning; past or current school reports; portfolios of work requiring academic skills; curriculum-based assessments; and past or current individual standardized test scores of academic achievement. If an intellectual, sensory, neurological, or motor disorder is suspected, the clinical evaluation for a specific learning disorder should also include methods appropriate for these disorders (American Psychiatric Association, 2013).

Thus, the comprehensive assessment will involve professionals with expertise in specific learning disorder and psychological/cognitive assessment, among which there may be a speech-language pathologist, a psychopedagogue, a neuropsychologist, a child and adolescent psychiatrist or a child neurologist, and an occupational therapist who performs sensory processing disorder assessment.

Other Conditions Frequent in the Office of the Child Behavior-Analytic Therapist

In addition to the three frameworks described above, several others can also be cited. Among them are:

- Eating disorders: these are conditions that already make us think of the need for a minimum team composed of a psychotherapist, psychiatrist, and nutritionist, in addition to close contact with the clinician/pediatrician to help with possible clinical complications that the eating disorder can generate. Other professionals can also make up the team in order to enhance and make the work possible, such as a family therapist, physical educator (to establish a healthy relationship

between the patient and physical activity), or even professionals who do not seem to be involved in the health area, such as a *personal stylist*, who could contribute to the process of reducing body dissatisfaction.
- Childhood obesity: although obesity is not included in DSM-5 as a psychiatric condition, there is a robust association between obesity and numerous psychiatric disorders (e.g., binge eating disorder, depressive disorder, bipolar disorder, and schizophrenia) (American Psychiatric Association, 2013). In addition to the professionals mentioned for eating disorders, the presence of a pediatric endocrinologist may be indispensable in the treatment of this increasingly common and harmful condition.
- Mood disorders (major depressive disorder, bipolar affective disorder) and anxiety disorders: besides the psychotherapist and the psychiatrist, other professionals can add important value to the treatment, such as the physical educator, the family therapist, and even a music teacher, through the increase of relaxing and naturally pleasurable activities.
- Various traumas: here the authors refer to specific situations that bring about important anxious symptoms and that, in a more acute instance, can be considered a posttraumatic stress disorder (although, with children, a complete diagnosis is not always reached). Assaults, fights, violent accidents, or sexual abuse involving the child or his/her family members may cause disruptive behaviors, insecure attachment, refusal to be alone, etc. These infinite so-called anxious responses are more easily treated by the psychotherapist when in conjunction with psychiatrists, pediatricians, and, sometimes, lawyers who point out to the family or affected party their legal rights in the situation and help them put into practice an action plan to prevent the recurrence of the situation, minimizing the psychological suffering of all involved.

Specificities of Teamwork

Assessment of the Case and Assembly of the Team

When parents seek the child behavior-analytic therapist, they may have already been referred by a physician (psychiatrist, pediatrician, neuropediatrician) or other health professionals. In this case, an attempt to work together with this professional is recommended, both for ethical reasons (e.g., professional courtesy) and for practical reasons, such as the fact that the professional has more information about the case and has a link with the family. In addition, it is assumed that whoever recommends the clinical behavior analysis for children, in his evaluation, considered that the therapy would be useful in improving the quality of life of that child, so taking this evaluation into account is an important step in the initial functional analysis.

In addition to the data brought by the evaluation of other professionals already treating the case, the initial evaluation work of the clinical behavior analyst for children is based on the collection of data with family/caregivers and with the children themselves (Silvares & Gongora, 1998; and Chap. 6 of this book). The information that will make the therapist aware of the need for a team is varied, ranging from functionalities that seem to have a phylogenetic etiology (genetic syndromes (e.g., children with syndromic features), atypical neurodevelopment (e.g., history of neurodevelopmental delay, impaired social interaction, stereotyped behaviors), epilepsy, ADHD, and other conditions) as for those that appear to have been modeled and maintained by ontogeny and culture (behavioral excesses and deficits – anxious, depressive, obsessive, and/or compulsive patterns; food refusal, restriction, or overeating; social and academic difficulties). It is essential to understand that the body functions as a whole and that behavior is multidetermined, and, therefore, its etiology can be found in different points of a continuum of the three levels of selection (Tourinho, 2012).

The invitation of a new professional to the case will happen if the therapist believes that the intervention will be beneficial to the progress of the case and if it will expand the child's repertoire in a way that clinical behavior analysis for children would not achieve with its tools or would not do so well or at the same speed as the chosen professional. Sometimes, the team may be assembled or even integrated by new professionals during the course of treatment. This will vary with the refinement of the interdisciplinary assessment of the case, since it does not take place only at the beginning of the sessions but remains longitudinally until discharge. It is important for the clinical behavior analyst for children to be aware of the responsibility in their hands when evaluating a child: based on a correct evaluation, team building, and treatment, they have the power to perform an early intervention that may prevent possible suffering during adolescence or adult life. Therefore, as previously mentioned, it is necessary for this professional to be aware of the functioning of the body as a whole, as well as the environment in which it is developing, both in sociocultural and biological terms (Peruzzolo et al., 2014), or even epigenetic (nutritional, digestive and excretory functioning, exposure to pathogens, etc.) (Jablonka & Lamb, 2010).

For example, children with oppositional, defiant, hyperactive, and/or inattentive patterns may have a chance to be less involved in alcohol and drug abuse and other antisocial behaviors in adulthood if they receive appropriate interdisciplinary treatment. For this, a team must be assembled that can look at all the demands of the child and manage their behavior and that of their families based on a common understanding of the functions of each response and the neurophysiological functioning of the client. Only then the team will be successful in the intervention with the child and in parental guidance, which should be ostensive and come from all professionals, consistently and coherently with the formulation of the case, each one respecting their area of expertise.

Other variables should also be analyzed when it comes time to assemble a team for a specific case. For example, the frequency, magnitude, and degree of the client's suffering in a certain area of his life may indicate to the therapist with which professional it is necessary to work. Issues such as the financial condition of the family also influence the invitation of one or more professionals to compose the team concomitantly or if it is necessary to first perform the interdisciplinary work with one and wait until discharge to enter the third.

Other Advantages of Teamwork

As previously explained, the main advantage of interdisciplinary team care is that, with the formulation of the case, there is a (or several) common objective(s) of the team, and, therefore, each professional will apply different treatments starting from their own reaches, to reach the expected final result.

When professionals integrate the technical knowledge of their areas, the tendency is that each one's work is optimized. For example, the clinical behavior analyst for children, having repeated measurements of his weekly sessions with the child, can access relevant information on the effect of prescribed psychiatric medications on the client's repertoire. Thus, the psychiatrist's work also interferes greatly with that of the clinical behavior analysis for children, since the use of drugs is an important independent environmental variable in reducing psychiatric symptoms and the effectiveness of certain reinforcers (McKim & Hancock, 2013). Any behavioral activation procedure, for example, established by clinical behavior analysis for children, will be more effective in a child with depressive symptoms who is receiving adequate drug treatment and, therefore, has his neuronal reward system functioning sufficiently so that the consequences of his responses have a reinforcing function (Stein et al., 1993).

Limitations and Difficulties of Teamwork

Interdisciplinary teamwork is not such a common reality in the Brazilian child behavior-analytic clinic. Such limitation is due to several factors, such as insistence on multidisciplinary approach, prejudice of clinical behavior analyst for children with the use of medications and techniques that are not within its scope, little appreciation of therapy by psychiatrists, little availability for team discussions, etc.

It is also common for professionals who refer to clinical behavior analysis for children, especially psychiatrists, to have difficulty interacting in an interdisciplinary group, seeking to maintain leadership in the group, and understanding therapy as a "conversation to calm the client down" while the medication takes effect. On the other hand, there is also the lack of knowledge by many psychologists of the importance of psychiatric medication in complex cases, sometimes leading to a competition between psychologist and psychiatrist about which of the two treatments is, in fact, being effective. A properly applied interdisciplinary approach breaks this prejudice: with evaluation and objectives being common to the team, successes are also celebrated as a team.

The lack of availability for team discussions may also stem from the routine of the health professionals involved, who tend to work many hours a week in assistance and devote little time to studies, case formulation, visits to schools, and finally, to teamwork. It is believed that an adequate and effective treatment in mental health requires that professionals dedicate themselves to the cases also in times outside the office, which would include conversations with team members, face-to-face or even virtual, for monitoring, discussion, and evolution of the chosen treatment.

Conclusion

The authors conclude that interdisciplinary care in children's clinical practice is possible and desirable, although difficult to implement. Complex family patterns, atypical neuronal functioning, epigenetic alterations changing sensitivities, and reinforcers are all variables relevant to child care and that result in excesses and behavioral *deficits that are* even more difficult to manage if the clinical behavior analyst for children is alone in this endeavor.

The intensity of the symptoms presented and the extent to which the child can deal with certain feelings/impulse control when given adequate support and contingencies are important factors to direct referral to a child and adolescent psychiatrist or child neurologist. The occurrence of demands/difficulties to be worked on that go beyond the scope of clinical behavior analyst for children also calls for the entry of more professionals in the treatment.

The analysis of each case will determine the team to be recruited, always taking into account the frameworks that usually require the entry of several professionals, the cost/benefit of the entry of each of them, and the availability and openness that they present for interdisciplinary work.

Among the numerous difficulties of interdisciplinary work, we can highlight the lack of awareness of the importance of this approach, the lack of availability of professionals, and the "dispute" regarding the degree of importance of the role of each professional to decide who will guide the best path to be followed.

The authors urge behavior analysts to get out of this interprofessional "scythe fight," as well as to be careful to identify which cases are more complex and will require a greater dedication outside the period of care. Even when the team does not yet function in an integrated manner, it is clinical behavior analyst for children's role, with all its knowledge about the multidetermination of human behavior and the pragmatism typical of radical behaviorism, to ignore the "ego squabbles" and continue inviting the professionals on the team to have a different posture focused on the well-being of the child being cared for.

References

American Psychiatric Association. (2013). *Diagnostic and statistical manual of mental disorders* (5th ed.) https://doi-org.ezproxy.frederick.edu/10.1176/appi.books.9780890425596

Battista, C., Evans, T. M., Ngoon, T. J., Chen, T., Chen, L., Kochalka, J., & Menon, V. (2018). Mechanisms of interactive specialization and emergence of functional brain circuits supporting cognitive development in children. *Science of Learning, 10*, 1–11. https://doi.org/10.1038/s41539-017-0017-2

Choi, B. C. K., & Pak, A. W. P. (2006). Multidisciplinarity, interdisciplinarity and transdisciplinarity in health research, services, education and policy: 1. Definitions, objectives, and evidence of effectiveness. *Clinical and Investigative Medicine, 29*, 351–364.

Hood, B. M. (1995). Shifts of visual attention in the human infant: A neuroscientific approach. *Advances in Infancy Research, 9*, 163–216.

Jablonka, E., & Lamb, M. J. (2010). *Evolução em quatro dimensões: DNA, comportamento e a história de vida*. Companhia das Letras.

Johnson, M. H. (1990). Cortical maturation and the development of visual attention in early infancy. *Journal of Cognitive Neuroscience, 2*, 81–95.

Martins Filho, A. J., & Martins, A. C. F. (2012). A complexidade da Infância: balanço de uma década das pesquisas com crianças apresentadas na ANPEd/Brasil. In L. Dornelles & N. Fernandes (Eds.), *Perspectivas sociológicas e educacionais em estudos da criança: as marcas das dialogicidades luso-brasileiras*. Centro de Investigação em Estudos da Criança, Universidade do Minho.

McKim, W. A., & Hancock, S. D. (2013). *Drugs & behavior: An introduction to behavioral pharmacology*. Pearson.

Morrow, R. L., Garland, E. J., Wright, J. M., Maclure, M., Taylor, S., & Dormuth, C. R. (2012). Influence of relative age on diagnosis and treatment of attention-deficit/hyperactivity disorder in children. *CMAJ, 184*(7), 755–762. https://doi.org/10.1503/cmaj.111619

Nowakowsk, R. S., & Hayes, N. L. (2012). Overview of early brain development: Linking genetics to brain structure. In W. Baker, A. Benasich, & R. H. Fitch (Eds.), *Developmental dyslexia: Early precursors, neurobehavioral markers, and Biological Substrates*. Brookes Publishing.

Palkhivala, A. (2010). How the environment shapes the brain. *Bulletin on Early Childhood Development, 9*, 3.

Papalia, D. E., Olds, S. W., & Feldman, R. D. (2009). *Desenvolvimento Humano*. McGraw-Hill Interamericana do Brasil Ltda.

Peruzzolo, D. L., Estivalet, K. M., Mildner, A. R., & Silveira, M. C. (2014). Participação da Terapia Ocupacional na equipe do Programa de Seguimento de Prematuros Egressos de UTINs. *Caderno de terapia ocupacional da UFSCar, 22*, 151–161.

Schore, J., & Schore, A. (2008). Modern attachment theory: The central role of affect regulation in development and treatment. *Clinical Social Work Journal, 36*, 9–20. https://doi.org/10.1007/s10615-007-0111-7

Shonkoff, J. P., & Phillips, D. A. (2000). *From neurons to neighborhoods: The science of early childhood development*. National Academy Press.

Silvares, E. F. M., & Gongora, M. A. N. (1998). *Psicologia Clínica Comportamental: A Inserção da Entrevista com Adultos e Crianças*. Edicon.

Stein, L., Xue, B. G., & Belluzzi, J. D. (1993). A cellular analogue of operant conditioning. *Journal of the Experimental Analysis of Behavior, 60*, 41–53.

Tourinho, E. Z. (2012). *Subjetividade e Relações comportamentais*. Centro Paradigma de Ciências do Comportamento.

Chapter 13
Functional Analysis of Interventions with Parents: Parental Orientation or Parent Training?

Giovana Del Prette, Caroline Drehmer Pilatti, Laura Malaguti Modernell, and Rodolfo Ribeiro Dib

This chapter aims to present a proposed definition and systematization of some aspects of the intervention with parents in Clinical Behavior Analysis for Children. Functional analysis will be used as the main thread of this systematization, covering the child's target behaviors, the classes of parenting practices, the clinician's assessment and intervention strategies, and the proposal of a definition of parent orientation and parent training.

Interventions with parents for behavior modification of children have existed for over five decades, constituting one of the first fields of applied research in behavior analysis. In the Journal of Applied Behavior Analysis (JABA), the first publication on the topic dates back to 1972, when Herbert and Baer presented the results of their research, entitled *Training parents as behavior modifiers: Self-recording of contingent attention* (Herbert & Baer, 1972). Child behavior-analytic clinicians have an explanatory system with concepts derived from laboratory research and a huge

---

G. Del Prette (✉) · C. D. Pilatti
Instituto de Psiquiatria do Hospital das Clínicas da Escola de Medicina da Universidade de São Paulo (IPq-USP), Child Adolescent and Adult Behavioral Analytic Clinical Association (ACACIA), São Paulo, Brazil
e-mail: caroline.pilatti@usp.br

L. M. Modernell
Faculty of Medicine, University of Geneva, Geneva, Switzerland

Child Adolescent and Adult Analytic-Behavioral Clinical Association (ACACIA), São Paulo, Brazil

R. R. Dib
Instituto de Psiquiatria do Hospital das Clínicas da Escola de Medicina da Universidade de São Paulo (IPq-USP), Child Adolescent and Adult Behavioral Analytic Clinical Association (ACACIA), São Paulo, Brazil

Paradigma - Center for Behavioral Sciences and Technology, São Paulo, Brazil

© The Author(s), under exclusive license to Springer Nature Switzerland AG 2022
A. S. U. Rossi et al. (eds.), *Clinical Behavior Analysis for Children*, https://doi.org/10.1007/978-3-031-12247-7_13

amount of systematized strategies in the literature, which enable them to directly assist children and/or intervene through their parents.

The main objective of the interventions with parents in Clinical Behavior Analysis for Children is the modification of parents' behaviors with a way of changing their interaction with the child and, in this way, promoting pro-social behaviors and reducing deviant behaviors (Kazdin, 1997). Behavioral interventions with parents start from the following assumptions: (1) the environment can produce, maintain, or intensify child behavior patterns; (2) the relationship with parents is a significant part of the child's environment; and, therefore, (3) children's behaviors can be modified by changing their parents' behaviors.

The assumption of influence of parental practices on children's behaviors does not mean that those (parental practices) are "the cause" of these (children's behaviors) or that they are "the only cause" and not even a "necessary or sufficient cause" (Kazdin, 1997). The behavioral explanation of any "cause" contemplates a complex network of influences of the three levels of selection – phylogenesis, ontogenesis, and culture (Skinner, 1953). Still, parents play a key role in child learning and development, for usually being the main attachment and affection figures (Troutman, 2015), for their decision-making power over many aspects of the child's life, and for the way they interact, evoking, reinforcing, and modeling behavioral patterns (Leijten et al., 2018). All these aspects meet the Skinnerian sense of the family's role as a controlling agency (Skinner, 1953).

Target Behaviors of the Child

In this chapter, we will start from the terminology and classification of the child's target behaviors proposed by Forehand and McMahon (2003): "OK behaviors" and "non-OK behaviors." According to the authors, non-OK behaviors are those which should decrease in frequency, and OK behaviors are all the others, which could or should happen more frequently, so that the sum of the two classes would correspond to the totality of the child's behaviors.

Forehand and McMahon's (2003) definition of OK behavior broadens the clinician's gaze and intervention to everything the child does, avoiding the polarization that restricts target behaviors based on opposing patterns (e.g., obey versus disobey). It is also an alternative to other value-judgmental terms (e.g., "appropriate" and "inappropriate" behaviors) and avoids any confusion with the lay use of the term "behavior problem" attributed mostly to children who "misbehave."

The delimitation of which behaviors will be considered OK or not OK by the clinician is done through an idiosyncratic functional analysis, that is, differentiated for each child seen. It is expected that every child presents behaviors that can be evaluated as OK and others as not OK. It is the deficits and excesses, respectively, in one and the other class, that can bring damage to their relationships and development in various spheres, such as affective, playful, intellectual, interpersonal, intrapersonal, and moral. In this sense, some classes of children's OK behaviors may be especially important, such as social and academic skills (Del Prette & Del Prette, 2005). Other behaviors are more evidently not OK because they cause harm to others, such as physical aggression (Patterson et al., 1992). Still others have less noticeable immediate consequences, but may compromise the child's development and be related to mental disorders in childhood, such as the use of tablets and mobile phones (Twenge & Campbel, 2018).

Finally, modifying the original definition by Forehand and McMahon (2003), in this chapter, we will characterize OK and non-OK behaviors from a triple contingency analysis and not only from the child's response. For example, instead of "disobeying parents" being a non-OK behavior, it would be defined as (a) characteristics of the command given by the parents (antecedent), (b) the disobedience (response), and (c) how the parents deal with the disobedience (consequences). That is, the entire contingency should happen less, not just the child's response. Thus, the criterion of increased or decreased frequency meets the definition of reinforcement, already specifying that there is a problem in the whole contingency, not just in what the child does. This inevitably leads us to the analysis of the behaviors of the individuals who participate in this contingency – in this case, the parents.

Target Behaviors of Parents

Although the very concept of behavior as an interaction between organism and environment justifies the insertion of parents in the therapy of their children, the rationale for including parents in the clinical behavior analysis for children may vary among treatments for different childhood disorders. For example, the insertion of parents into therapy for children with disobedience and aggression problems is primarily related to modifying coercive cycles of interaction that intensify "disruptive" behaviors (Patterson et al., 1992). In therapy for children with anxiety problems, family accommodation that maintains the anxious pattern would be the primary target of intervention with parents (Lebowitz et al., 2019). For children diagnosed with autism spectrum disorder (ASD), the insertion of parents would be primarily related to the need to maintain and generalize the skills taught in the individual treatment of their children (Brookman-Frazee et al., 2009).

Consistent with our previous proposal regarding the definition of OK and not OK behaviors, and with the therapeutic implication of changing the terms of contingency that correspond to the parents' responses, we will propose here an analysis of parenting practices that may be applicable regardless of the reason for referring the child to psychotherapy. In this analysis – and in the proposal that follows – parental behaviors are organized into three main classes: (a) precurrent behaviors, (b) contingency arrangement behaviors, and (c) behaviors in the interaction with the child.

Parental Precurrent Behaviors

Precurrent behaviors are private and public responses that produce or alter discriminative stimuli and, as consequences, affect the probability of occurrence of subsequent responses from the same individual (Baum, 1994; Skinner, 1969). In the case of parenting practices, we are referring to various parental behaviors that produce discriminative stimuli that influence the probability of occurrence of (a) new precurrent behaviors, of (b) contingency arrangement behaviors, and (c) how they interact with the child.

In a behavioral chain, it is possible that the parents' first precursors are the private responses that put themselves under control of the child's behavior or of one or more aspects of this behavior. This could be called "perceiving," "paying attention," and "observing" (cf. Skinner, 1953; Skinner, 1957; Strapasson & Dittrich, 2008). The individual himself (mother/father) can be a stimulus for the precursor, as in the case of self-observation, which would be equivalent to parents observing themselves and how they are a stimulus for the child's responses.

Behaviors that aid in problem-solving and decision-making can also be considered precursors (Rodrigues & Linares, 2014). At a private level, this is equivalent to what we usually call "reasoning", "deducing", "imagining", "analyzing", "hypothesizing", and so on (Baum, 1994). In the context of parenting practices, when parents analyze the child's behaviors, they are behaving in ways that alter the likelihood that they will act in one direction or another to deal with those behaviors. The parents' public behaviors of seeking and obtaining information (such as when reading a book, asking for advice, listening to a clinician), writing notes, reporting the child's behaviors, or even the act of empirically testing a hypothesis are also pre-occurring.

The parents' degree of expertise in one or more of these precurrent behaviors may influence – compromising or contributing to – all the next steps that would culminate in an effective management of their children's behavior. Ultimately, deficits in parents' repertoire of precurrent behaviors may be part of the maintenance of the child's behavior patterns (Briegel et al., 2019), making it harder for parents to help the child, or even biasing the clinical's analysis and interventions based on the parents' report.

Precurrent behaviors should be part of the clinician's contingency analysis (Rodrigues & Linares, 2014). In the case of intervention with parents at Clinical Behavior Analysis for Children, this means assessing and intervening on the precursors so as to lead parents to improve their perception, self-observation, analyses, hypotheses, use of notes and diaries, search and systematization of information, empirical tests and reports on the child's behavior.

Parental Contingency Arrangement Behaviors

We are calling contingency arrangement behaviors the parental practices that occur under control of discriminative stimuli produced by precurrent behaviors (described above) and that produce, as a consequence, temporary or prolonged changes in the child's physical and/or social environment. We will exclude here the parents' behaviors in direct interaction with the child, since they will be addressed in the next item. Next, we present a functional analysis of the contingency arrangement behaviors, suggesting some examples of parental responses and the expected consequences on the child's behavior.

The examples listed in Table 13.1 illustrate that contingency arrangement behaviors include a large implementation set of parental decisions that affect children's behaviors. The first and most obvious effect on the child is to define the limits of his action within the possibilities arranged by the parents. In other words, certain behaviors of the child are only possible because of this arrangement, and, additionally, other behaviors become impossible.

Table 13.1 Discriminative stimuli, parental responses, and consequences in parental contingency arrangement behaviors

Discriminative stimuli	Answers	Consequences
Products of discriminative stimuli produced by parents' precurrent behaviors	Parents arrange temporary and/or prolonged contingencies in the child's physical and/or social environment	Producing temporary or prolonged changes in the child's physical and/or social environment that impacts on child's behavior
Perceive, observe, reflect, analyze, seek information, systematize notes, report about the child to a listener, test hypotheses, etc.	Organize routine and decide schedules	Child behaves within the possibilities of that routine and schedule
	Enrolling in a particular school	Child attends the chosen school daily
	Adapting the child's physical space	Child acts within the possibilities of that space
	Providing or preventing access to certain toys, objects, and food	Child plays with toys, uses objects, and eats available food - and not other options
	Promote meetings with other children and family members	Child has access to interact with these children and family members
	Choosing types of tours and trips	Child has access to the contexts provided by these outings and trips
	Alter various motivating operations deprivation and satiation	Changes various probabilities of child responses and value of reinforcers

The contingency arrangement is an important part of parenting practices, since parents are the ones who have the greatest power of decision about macrocontingencies in the lives of their children. The choice of school, activity schedules, types of toys, food, outings, trips, and meetings are some examples that ultimately define what characterizes and what does not characterize the child's daily life.

This group of parenting practices also includes the arrangement of day-to-day microcontingencies with the child. This happens when parents remove competing stimuli and/or bring closer stimuli that set the occasion for an expected behavior. Turning off the lights and turning off the TV moments before bedtime, for example, removes competing stimuli with those that would evoke the response of going to bed, while making children's books available near the bed could evoke the child's response of lying down and read, thus approaching the subsequent response of going to sleep.

Modifying motivational operations is also an arrangement of contingencies (e.g., McGinnis et al., 2010), making a behavior more or less likely by establishing or abolishing, respectively, the reinforcing value of the consequences it produces. The length of the interval that a child goes without eating, for example, may alter the likelihood that she will accept the salad at lunch time. The length of the interval that he/she goes without attention can impact the probability of trying to get this attention from her parents in ways that are not OK but highly effective, even when also being punished. Deprivation of food, drink, and sleep; prolonged exposure to auditory and visual stimulation (such as watching TV); scarcity of stimuli (which we would call boredom); restriction of physical space; and deprivation of social interaction are examples of motivational operations that alter emotional states (as in the case of irritability) and the probability of non-OK behaviors. In this way, the contingency arrangement behaviors also includes the way parents manage motivational operations of the child's behavior.

The arrangement of macro- and microcontingencies does not infallibly determine the child's behavior; it only makes it physically possible or impossible, more or less likely. The contingencies arranged by parents can bring solutions, but also problems and challenges. In the intervention with parents, the clinical behavior analyst must obtain the necessary information about which are the macro- and microcontingencies arranged by parents, to analyze how they may be contributing or not to the occurrence of OK and non-OK behaviors of the child. From this, the professional can help parents to arrange new contingencies that contribute to the increase of OK behaviors and the reduction of non-OK behaviors. However, intervening on parent's contingency arrangement behaviors is usually not enough to change the child's behavior, being also necessary the intervention on how parents interact with the child.

Parental Behaviors in Their Interaction with the Child

Contingency analysis of parent-child interaction allows the clinician to systematize hypotheses about how parents' actions may function as antecedents and/or consequences for the child's OK and non-OK responses (and vice versa). For didactic purposes, we schematize below three patterns of contingencies, not mutually exclusive, in which the parent-child interaction may contribute to the increase of non-OK responses by the child and/or the decrease of OK responses: (1) coercive cycle, (2) excesses in reinforcing child's non-OK responses, and (3) deficits in reinforcing child's OK responses.

The first pattern of contingencies in Table 13.2, "coercive cycle," corresponds to coercive ways in which parents interact with the child in an attempt to make him/her behave in an OK way and/or to reduce his/her non-OK behaviors (Patterson et al., 1992). It is characterized first by the presence of parent's aversive stimulation as antecedent of child's behavior, such as threats, criticism, or lectures. Faced with this, there are two possible outcomes for the child. First, the child responds in an OK manner and thereby avoids the aversive situation (negative reinforcement). In the second, the child responds in a non-OK manner, and the parents intensify the aversive stimulation or apply some new punishment (such as sanctions, physical aggression, loss of privileges, and humiliation).

We call this pattern the "coercive cycle" because parent and child function as aversive stimuli to each other and the actions of both are sometimes punished and sometimes negatively reinforced. The child's non-OK response is an aversive stimulus for the parent, and the use of threats, criticism, and lectures is reinforced by intermittently producing child's OK responses. When the child repeats the non-OK response, this aggravates the aversive stimulus until it is suppressed and/or evokes an OK response, in both cases negatively reinforcing the parent's pattern.

However, in the period when the parents threaten, criticize, lecture, or punish the child, the interaction itself can also function as positive reinforcement for non-OK behavior, since provides to the child attention and care, even if in the form of recriminations. When this happens, there is an intersection between the class "coercive cycle" and the second class in Table 13.2 of "excesses in reinforcing child's non-OK responses."

Table 13.2 Contingency analysis of parental behaviors in the interaction with the child: coercive cycle, excesses in reinforcing child's non-OK responses, and *deficits* in reinforcing child's OK responses

Contingency pattern	Parental actions functioning as antecedents to Child's responses	Child's responses	Parental actions functioning as consequences to child's responses
1. Coercive cycle	1. Parent's coercive behavior as aversive stimuli for child's OK or non-OK responses	1. Child's OK responses	1. Child avoids punishment (negative reinforcement avoiding)
		1 and 2. Child's non-OK responses	1 and 2. Parents continue or intensify cohertion (Positive and negative punishment)
2. Excesses in reinforcing child's non-OK responses	2. Parent's provide excessive discriminative stimuli for child's non-OK responses		1 and 2. Parents reacts are More likely positive reinforcement, in greater magnitude, duration, and contiguity
3. *Deficits in reinforcing* child's OK responses	3. Parent's provide few discriminative stimuli for child's OK responses	3. Child's OK responses	3. Parents reacts are less likely positive reinforcement, in smaller magnitude and duration, and not very contiguous

These excesses correspond to parents' actions that, firstly, amplify the opportunities (discriminative stimuli) for the occurrence of the child's non-OK responses. As an example, we can cite the exaggerated quantity and bad topography of orders that some parents give throughout the day, or even questions and comments that tend to "remind" the child of his/her non-OK behaviors ("Are you really telling mom the truth?" "Let's see if this time you won't throw the food on the floor!).

Then, in the face of non-OK responses by the child, the consequences given by the parents may function both as positive reinforcement (maintaining the child's non-OK pattern) and also as punishment (by the aversive component), again intersecting with the coercive cycle pattern. Positive reinforcement occurs especially when there is greater likelihood, magnitude, duration, and contiguity of parental consequences in the face of child's non-OK response, than in the face of the child's OK's. In other words, parents may be more likely to blurt out some reaction when the child is yelling than when he/she is in silence. A lecture when the child messes up is usually much longer than a positive comment when the child completes his homework. Parents will probably react immediately if the child starts scribbling on the walls, but not so immediately if he/she starts putting a puzzle together. Anyway, parents can be pretty consistent in inadvertently teaching their child non-OK responses.

Finally, the third pattern of contingencies in Table 13.2 are deficits in the reinforcement of the child's OK responses. In this sense, the clinician also assesses whether there are important skills that the parents do not have (in the sense of never having learned them), whether they do have but are infrequently, or whether they have the skills but they are somehow functionally ineffective in increasing the child's OK and reducing non-OK behaviors.

Regarding the antecedents, the parents may provide little opportunity for the child's OK responses, which can happen in several ways. One of the ways is by "underutilizing" the natural daily situations and the child's abilities, for example, by not including the child in the household activities, by doing for the child what he/she could do by him/herself, or by responding for the child in a conversation with someone else. Another form of reduced opportunity is when the parents' actions do not function as discriminative stimuli for the child's OK responses because of the topography of these actions. For example, orders that are confusing, too long, or given when they are far away from the child may make it difficult for being accomplished. Finally, if there is little reinforcing consequences for child's OK responses, then parental actions, even if topographically "correct," are not functionally established as evoking child's OK responses.

Deficits in providing reinforcing consequences for child's OK responses occurs when these consequences may be less likely, of lower magnitude and duration, and less contiguous to these OK responses than to the child's non-OK responses. In addition, topography again may be important for functioning as a reinforcing consequence. For example, vague praise such as "well done" and "congratulations" and comments with embedded criticism such as "I like it, but why don't you always do it like that?" or said in a mechanical way, without vocal intonation and without eye contact, may not reinforce anything and may even be aversive to the child.

In short, based on the functional analysis of the parents' interaction with the child before and throughout the intervention sessions, the clinician identifies excesses and deficits of the parents reppertoire that could play a role in maintaining the child's problem. The identification of the type of deficit (cf. Gresham, 2013) may be important to guide the clinician's intervention strategies to, respectively, teach parents new skills, promote an increase in the frequency of existing skills, or modify aspects such as topography, contiguity, magnitude, and consistency to improve their functionality.

Assessment and Intervention Strategies with Parents

Good behavioral treatment with parents should be based on functional analysis of behavior and not only on the diagnostic of specific symptoms (Chronis et al., 2004). Functional analysis enables the clinician to know how to lead parents to modify antecedents and consequences of the child's behaviors. The functional analysis covers – or should cover – not only the child's target behaviors and parental practices but also the clinician's own behaviors, i.e., hypotheses about how their interventions in session will function as antecedents and consequences to modify parents' responses that, in turn, produce changes on children's responses (Del Prette, 2017). All this information is important for the clinician to make the best decisions about how to structure the sessions with parents, which strategies to use, and how to assess the impact of their interventions on both parents' and children's behaviors.

Although these aspects would be generally accepted by clinicians, a comparison between four important manuals of behavioral intervention with parents in the literature, conducted by Del Prette (2017), showed that there are substantial differences between the proposals, starting with the use of other explanatory models in addition to behavior analysis, which may be reflected in the other differences found in this study. Differences were also found in the definition of the child's and parents' target behaviors and, mainly, in the selection of assessment and intervention strategies, how to use them, and the proportion of session time devoted to them.

Despite the differences between the proposals, as described in the manuals, the international literature usually refers to all behavioral interventions with parents as "parent training" (e.g. Barkley, 1996; Dailey et al., 2017; Kazdin, 2008; Sonuga-Barke et al., 2013). In Brazil, the literature uses both the term "parental training" and "parental orientation" (as in Coelho & Murta, 2007; Marinho, 1999; Pinheiro et al., 2006), the latter being the most frequent/usual among Brazilian clinical behavior analyst for children to name their practice.

In our literature searches for this chapter, we did not find a unique and clear distinction between the terms "parent orientation" and "parent training" nor between the practices of the clinician to which they refer. Therefore, we will propose below a definition of the terms "orient" and "train," based on the etymology of these words, in order to identify the assessment and intervention strategies with parents most relevant to the definition of one and the other and, based on these strategies, proceed to a functional analysis of the clinician's actions in each of these two general classes of intervention.

Parental Orientation Interventions

The word "orient"[1] comes from the Latin *oriens, entis*, meaning "oriental; orient, part of the sky where the sun rises." "Orient" as a noun, therefore, originally meant "act or effect of orienting or directing toward the east." From Latin to French ("orienter") and to Portuguese (orientar), we have the current definition of "to show the direction; to direct, guide, forward, guide; to orient someone in the right direction" (Houaiss & Villar, 2009).

Orienting, while synonym of "indicating a path" means, therefore, suggesting a possibility of action, which may or may not be adopted by who requests the guidance. Also, it will be executed only a posteriori, that is, in some moment after the interaction between who guives and who receives the orientation. For example, a lost person can ask for help to someone on the street, and this person, in turn, indicates a path to reach the destination (often, for this, it is necessary to ask more questions, describe, explain, etc.), and, as a consequence, the lost person has new information, which may or may not be used later.

Drawing a parallel with this example, we would say that in parental orientation is (a) the clinician collects information based primarily on verbal discriminative stimuli emitted by parents in the session about the child's OK and non-OK behaviors (reports, analyses, responses to inventories, etc.), (b) the clinician's responses are antecedents or consequences to the parents' reports and analyses and indicate a "path" to be followed, and (c) he/she produces, as consequences in the session itself, changes in the parents' verbal behavior (modifications in the report, reflections, confirmations that they will try to follow the indicated path) that may correspond to future changes outside the session. The clinician's actions related to giving parental orientations may include asking for reports and reflections (as antecedents to the parents' reports), providing explanations, empathizing, formulating analyses, approving or disagreeing, making recommendations, and proposing homework assignments (as consequences of the parents' reports).

The attempt to follow the orientation is made *outside* the session, and, therefore, as a rule, the child is not present in the sessions (or, if he or she is, the main interventions are still focused on future follow-up). The absence of the child from the sessions makes it unfeasible to observe parent-child interaction as an evaluation measure, but it can be compensated for by requesting filming outside the office,

---

[1] While in Brazil the word "orientation" is used, the English literature usually uses the term "counseling" to refer to the practice of the "counselor," including parental counseling. *Counseling* is the verb form of the noun *counsel*, meaning "to give advice, warning or recommendation." Therefore, we consider counseling to be synonymous with orienting and will refer only to "parental orientation."

applying inventories, and observing the child individually in clinical behavior analysis for children sessions.

In terms of classes of parenting practices, parental orientation enables the clinician to directly access (via observation) only the change of some precursor behaviors, such as reporting, listening to the information, analysis and advice, and doing their own analysis. If parents attempt to follow the guidance, the orientations received would function as verbal supplementation evoking responses outside the session according to the guided content. But the clinician has little or no access to and control over *whether* and *how* parents will behave in the guided direction, altering contingency arrangement practices and interaction with the child, nor whether this will be effective in reducing non-OK behaviors and increasing OK behaviors.

Role-playing is a widely used technique that could bring, with limitations, the direct access to parenting skills within the session. It is usually referred to as an opportunity for parents to practice skills in session by simulating, with the clinician, the interaction that should occurr with the child outside the session (Thompson & Laver-Bradubury, 2013). Role-playing is suggested in intervention manuals with parents, but not always combined with feedback, modeling, and/or role-modeling (Del Prette, 2017). In fact, role-playing allows clinicians to observe the parents' performance in a simulated situation, but, as there is no access to the real parent-child interaction, it would not be an intervention on truly parents' behavior (including antecedents, responses, and natural consequences provided by the child) but on their responses in the session.

Among the four intervention manuals with parents analyzed by Del Prette (2017), the assessment and intervention strategies of three of them would correspond more appropriately to the definition of parental orientation, even though they receive the label of "parent training": *Defiant children: A clinician's manual for assessment and parent training* (Barkley, 1996), *Incredible Years* (Webster-Stratton & Reid, 2012), and *New Forest Parenting Programme* (Thompson & Laver-Bradubury, 2013). In Barkley's (1996) program, the main strategy of intervention is by presenting and discussing the content with the parents, who receive homework assignments between sessions, with role-playing being optional and, according to the author, dispensable. In Webster-Stratton and Reid (2012), the sessions are composed of approximately 25% videomodelling, 15% didactic teaching of the proposed skills, and 60% group discussion and support (cf. Forehand & McMahon, 2003). Finally, the sessions in Thompson and Laver-Bradubury's (2013) program take place in the family's home and in the presence of the child, but the child participates only in the final moments of one fifth of the sessions, so that the clinician can observe the parent-child interaction (without intervening) and provide feedback in the next session. Again, most of the time, the therapist's strategies are based on didactic explanations and discussions, with parent-clinician role-playing if necessary.

Parental Training Interventions

The word "train" comes from the Latin traxinare, past tense of traho, which also means "to pull" (Etymonline, 2019). From traxinare was derived the word traisner in Old French (traîsner), which means "to pull, to drag, to carry with you, to take someone by force." Traxinare was also derived into Medieval English as train, meaning "to drag" (and therefore, when hence steam engines were invented, received the name train). The term was incorporated into the Portuguese language as "treinar," meaning "to exercise; to perform a certain activity regularly" and "to submit to training, to train, to habituate," also becoming used as a sports word.

Training, meaning exercising regularly in order to "drag" toward the final objective, requires preparing conditions that lead the individual to practice in the presence of the trainer, so that he/she can observe, measure progress, and continuously intervene during this practice. A physical trainer, for example, prepares exercises, instructs, demonstrates how to do them, observes the person practicing, makes adjustments and gives feedback on their performance, and measures the performance to progressively increase the difficulty/complexity of the exercises, until the individual reaches the expected training.

Drawing a parallel with parent training, we would say that training requires the clinician to plan the structure of the sessions in advance in order to bring the parenting practices into the clinic, which includes the child's responses as antecedents and consequences to the parent's responses and these as antecedents and consequences to the child's responses. This means that the presence of the child in the session is the minimum requirement for training to take place. Thus, in parental training: (a) the clinician the parental practices in the parent-child interaction in session are the mainly discriminative stimuli for the clinician's analysis and interventions; (b) the clinician's responses are antecedents or consequences that affect this interaction, and (c) the immediate consequences these clinician's responses produce are changes in parental practices and in the child's target behaviors toward the final goal, observed and measured in their interaction in session.

The clinician's responses include, first, structuring the sessions with exercises or situations in session that should evoke the target behaviors of the parents and the child, making it possible to observe and measure them as the main measure of evaluation. The clinician's interventions take place on the parent-child interaction and may include giving instructions and modeling (as antecedents of the parents' actions), describing, approving, empathizing, disagreeing, analyzing, and giving continuous and immediate *feedback* (as consequences of the parents' actions). The clinician's interventions aim to evoke and model new parental responses that produce immediate changes in the child's response and, in turn, also naturally reinforce parental changes. Homework assignments are used as a way to promote the generalization, outside the clinic and to other situations, of a learning that has already begun in the session.

In parent training, the clinician can observe and intervene over the three classes of parenting practices presented in the previous section. The parents' precurrent behaviors – of perceiving, observing, describing, and analyzing – are based on stimuli present in the very session, which allows the clinician to verify and train the correspondence between stimuli and verbal responses. The clinician can teach microcontingency arrangements in the session itself, such as the choice of toys, organization and arrangement of the environment, and management of the intervals of child's attention deprivation. The clinician can also teach parenting skills in their interaction with the child.

Two examples of parent training manuals that include all the abovementioned elements are *Helping the Noncompliant Child* (Forehand & McMahon, 2003) and *Parent-Child Interaction Therapy* (Eyberg & Funderburk, 2011) for individual application and with the child's participation, respectively, in all or most sessions. Practicing exercises and playing in parent-child interaction should occupy most of the time of the sessions, allowing continuous observation, measurement, and modeling. During the rest of the session, the clinician presents the parents a new skill and analyzes the exercises practiced or the reports and notes on homework. These moments may also include strategies that we classify as parental orientation (including *role-playing*), but, in the meantime, the presence of the child continues to be used by the clinician to evoke target behaviors and teach parents how to manage them. Homework assignments consist of exercises identical to those practiced in session, aiming to generalize the interaction skills trained for everyday situations with the child, with worksheets for parents to record their performance.

In the functional analysis of the interventions described in the four manuals of intervention with parents, Del Prette (2017) concluded that the more effective the interventions (according to the meta-analysis of Sonuga-Barke et al., 2013 and the clinical trial of Abikoff et al., 2015), the greater the theoretical consistency of their proposals with the framework of behavior analysis in relation to the definition of child and parent target behaviors, the intervention strategies, and the forms of outcome assessment. Of the four manuals analyzed by Del Prette (2017), the intervention manualized in *Helping the Noncompliant Child* (Forehand & McMahon, 2003) was the one with the largest effect size (cf. Abikoff et al., 2015), being the only one built based only on the behavioral approach, whose assessment and intervention strategies were compatible with the definition of parent training that we proposed in this chapter.

In sum, the terms "orienting" and "training" have distinct meanings and correspond to different combinations of assessment and intervention strategies, acting on different processes of change. The clinician may choose between parental orientation and parent training but also mix strategies from one or the other practice. However, the functional analysis we have proposed on parent training suggests greater possibility of clinician control over all three classes of parenting practices. Since the parent-child interaction takes place under his eyes, the results of the intervention on this interaction also take place in the session itself and not only outside of it.

Final Considerations

In this chapter, we sought to describe the aspects that we consider relevant in a clinical intervention with parents, considering research results and the principles of behavior analysis. The analysis presented does not exhaust the possibilities but covers the main aspects related to the three main characters of the clinician's work with parents: the child, the parents, and the clinician. In all the points covered in our chapter, the functional analysis is considered a guide for the systematization of existing information in the literature and as a basis for the proposals and definitions suggested.

We hope that some of the hypotheses suggested in this chapter may be the object of future studies and that they expand Del Prette's (2017) analysis to other intervention manuals with proven effectiveness, comparing them in terms of the child's target behaviors, parenting practices, assessment and intervention strategies, and their correspondence with parental orientation or parent training. This is also justified as a resource to verify possible correlations with the results of research using programs based on one or another type of intervention. It is worth mentioning the importance of systematic reviews and meta-analyses considering the content of parenting intervention manuals for the comparison of interventions and not restricting themselves to the information summarized in research articles based on these manuals.

Notwithstanding the lack of a separate systematic review of the literature for orienting and training programmes, we understand from examining the literature cited that behavioral interventions really based on parent training strategies, as we define it, are likely to be an exception among behavioral interventions with parents in both brazilian and international literature. Even if there are other programs available, in addition to those mentioned here (Eyberg & Funderburk, 2011; Forehand & McMahon, 2003), it is possible that training constitutes a minority. In other words, most of the studies describing, comparing, or reviewing parenting interventions would be referring to interventions based on orientation strategies, including those referred to as training. In this case, there would still be much research to be done on the effect of interventions that manage antecedents and consequences of parenting practices in the face-to-face clinical context of parent-child interaction.

Transposing the subject of what interventions with parents are like to be used by clinicians in Clinical Behavior Analysis for Children in Brazil, the clinician's strategies are, as a rule, called "parental orientation" and in fact correspond to the act of orienting, as we defined in the chapter. In addition, sessions with parents usually occur sparsely (e.g., Conte & Regra, 2000), often becoming adjuncts to the child's weekly psychotherapy sessions. The choice for less frequent interventions with parents seems to contradict the premise that changes in parents' behaviors have been considered a key mechanism in producing changes in children's behavior (McMahon, 2015). This leads us to question why this format is maintained, despite the research evidence on the benefits of interventions with fathers. We can only hypothesize a few things.

A first hypothesis would be the very scarcity of alternatives to this model published in the literature, leading the clinician to learn only the practice of parental guidance. Another hypothesis is the perpetuation of a cultural practice, transmitted by the group, from generation to generation, via verbal behavior (cf. Baum, 1994). Thus, weekly sessions with the child and sporadic ones with parents, based on guidance strategies, would characterize a cultural practice of child psychotherapy (even independently of the approach) in Brazil.

We understand that both research and clinical practice still have a long way to go and, certainly, a challenge ahead: to modify this cultural practice, if this is necessary to achieve better results. Interventions with parents, when effective, alter contingencies not only in the service of the assisted individual but also toward a less coercive world, with less suffering, expressing our responsibility and professional commitment to changes oriented toward the good of the culture.

Enabling parents to promote behavioral changes in their children is to intervene between generations, which can extend beyond parents and children, because "the good of culture, like the good of others, also refers to others with this difference: they are the others of the future, our children and our grandchildren and the children and grandchildren of others who are our contemporaries" (Abib, 2001, p. 114). Changing the course of coercive cycles, getting parents to change the way they perceive and relate to their children while they are still children is ultimately acting today on the others of the future.

References

Abib, J. A. D. (2001). Teoria moral de Skinner e Desenvolvimento Humano. *Psicologia: Reflexão e Crítica, 14*(1), 107–117.

Abikoff, H. B., Thompson, M., Laver-Bradbury, C., Long, N., Forehand, R. L., Miller Brotman, L., Klein, R. G., Reiss, P., Huo, L., & Sonuga-Barke, E. (2015). Parent training for preschool ADHD: A randomized controlled trial of specialized and generic programs. *Journal of Child Psychology and Psychiatry, 56*(6), 618–631.

Barkley, R. A. (1996). *Defiant children: A clinician's manual for assessment and parent training*. The Guilford Press.

Baum, W. (1994). *Understanding behaviorism: Behavior, culture, and evolution*. Wiley-Blackwell.

Briegel, W., Greuel, J., Stroth, S., & Heinrichs, N. (2019). Parents' perception of their 2–10-year-old Children's contribution to the dyadic parent-child relationship in terms of positive and negative behaviors. *International Journal of Environmental Research and Public Health, 16*(7), 1123.

Brookman-Frazee, L., Vismara, L., Drahota, A., Stahmer, A., & Openden, D. (2009). Parent training interventions for children with autism spectrum disorders. In *Applied behavior analysis for children with autism spectrum disorders* (pp. 237–257). Springer.

Chronis, A. M., Chacko, A., Fabiano, G. A., Wymbs, B. T., & Pelham, W. E. (2004). Enhancements to the behavioral parent training paradigm for families of children with ADHD: Review and future directions. *Clinical Child and Family Psychology Review, 7*(1), 1–26.

Coelho, M. V., & Murta, S. G. (2007). Treinamento de pais em grupo: um relato de experiência. *Estudos de Psicologia, 24*(3), 333–341.

Conte, F. C. S., & Regra, J. A. G. (2000). A psicoterapia comportamental infantil: Novos aspectos. In E. M. F. Silvares (Ed.), *Estudos de caso em psicologia clínica comportamental infantil* (Vol. 1, pp. 79–136). Papirus.

Dailey, D., et al. (2017). Current best practice in the use of parent training and other behavioural interventions in the treatment of children and adolescents with attention deficit hyperactivity disorder. *Journal of Child Psychology and Psychiatry, 59*(9), 932–947.

Del Prette, G. (2017). *Adaptação e aplicação de um programa para Treinamento Parental Comportamental no tratamento de pré-escolares com Transtorno de déficit de atenção/hiperatividade. Relatório final de pós-doutorado*. Núcleo de Pesquisa em Neurodesenvolvimento e Saúde Mental, Instituto de Psiquiatria da Universidade de São Paulo. Orientador: Dr. Guilherme Vanoni Polanczyk.

Del Prette, Z. A. P., & Del Prette, A. (2005). Psicologia das Habilidades Sociais na infância: Teoria e prática. *Vozes*.

Etymolonline. (2019). https://www.etymonline.com/word/train

Eyberg, S. M., & Funderburk, B. W. (2011). *Parent-child interaction therapy protocol*. PCIT International.

Forehand, R. L., & McMahon, R. J. (2003). *Helping the noncompliant child: Family-based treatment for oppositional behavior*. Guilford Press.

Gresham, F. M. (2013). Análise do comportamento aplicada às Habilidades Sociais. In A. Del Prette & Z. A. P. Del Prette (Eds.), *Psicologia das Habilidades Sociais: Diversidade teórica e suas implicações* (3rd ed., pp. 18–66). USP.

Herbert, E. W., & Baer, D. (1972). Training parentes as behavior modifiers: Self-recording of contingent attention. *Journal of Applied Behavior Analysis, 5*(2), 139–149.

Houaiss, A. & Villar, M. S. (2009). *Dicionário Houaiss de Língua Portuguesa. Elaborado pelo Instituto Antônio Houaiss de Lexicografia e Banco de Dados da Língua Portuguesa S/C Ltda.* .

Kazdin, A. E. (1997). Parent management training: Evidence, outcomes and issues. *Journal of the American Academy of Child and Adolescent Psychiatry, 36*(10), 1349–1356.

Kazdin, A. E. (2008). *Parent management training: Treatment for oppositional, aggressive, and antisocial behavior in children and adolescents*. Oxford University Press.

Lebowitz, E. R., Marin, C., Martino, A., Shimshoni, Y., & Silverman, W. K. (2019). Parent-based treatment as efficacious as cognitive-behavioral therapy for childhood anxiety: A randomized noninferiority study of supportive parenting for anxious childhood emotions. *Journal of the American Academy of Child & Adolescent Psychiatry*. https://doi.org/10.1016/j.jaac.2019.02.014

Leijten, P., Gardner, F., Melendez-Torres, G. J., Knerr, W., & Overbeek, G. (2018). Parenting behaviors that shape child compliance: A multilevel meta-analysis. *PLoS One, 13*(10), e0204929.

Marinho, M. L. (1999). *Orientação de pais em grupo: intervenção sobre diferentes queixas comportamentais infantis*. Universidade de São Paulo.

McGinnis, M. A., Houchins-Jua'rez, N., McDaniel, J. L., & Kennedy, C. H. (2010). Abolishing and establishing operation analysis of social attention as positive reinforcement for problem behavior. *Journal of Applied Behavior Analysis, 43*, 119–123.

McMahon, R. J. (2015). *Parent management training interventions for preschool-age children. Encyclopedia on early childhood development*. Center of Excellence for Early Childhood Development.

Patterson, G., Reid, J., & Dishion, T. (1992). *Antisocial boys*. Castalia; Eugene.

Pinheiro, M. I. S., Haase, V. H., Del Prette, A., Amarante, C. L. D., & Del Prette, Z. A. P. (2006). Treinamento de habilidades sociais educativas para pais de crianças com problemas de comportamento. *Psicologia: Reflexão e Crítica, 19*(3), 407–414.

Rodrigues, B., & Linares, I. (2014). O manejo de precorrentes para a alteração de um processo de tomada de decisão. *Comportamento em foco, 3*, 263–268.

Skinner, B. F. (1953). *Science and human behavior*. Macmillan.

Skinner, B. F. (1957). *Verbal Behavior*. Appleton-Century-Crofts.

Skinner, B. F. (1969). *Contingencies of reinforcement: A theoretical analysis*. Appleton-century-crofts.

Sonuga-Barke, E. J., Brandeis, D., Cortese, S., Daley, D., Ferrin, M., Holtmann, M., Stevenson, J., Danckaerts, M., van der Oord, S., Döpfner, M., Dittmann, R. W., Simonoff, E., Zuddas, A., Banashewski, T., Buitelaar, J., & Coghill, D. (2013). Nonpharmacological interventions for ADHD: Systematic review and meta-analysis of randomized controlled trials of dietary and psychological treatments. *The American Journal of Psychiatry, 170*(3), 275–289.

Strapasson, B. A., & Dittrich, A. (2008). O conceito de prestar atenção para Skinner. *Psicologia: Teoria e Pesquisa [online], 24*(4), 519–526.

Thompson, M. J., & Laver-Bradubury, C. (2013). *New Forest parenting Programme: A timely, target and theoretically based intervention for children with ADHD difficulties: Na 8 week home based programme*. Notes for Therapists: Manual in press.

Troutman, B. (2015). *Integrating behaviorism and attachment theory in parent coaching*. Springer.

Twenge, J. M., & Campbel, W. K. (2018). Associations between screen time and lower psychological Well-being among children and adolescents: Evidence from a population-based study. *Preventive Medicine Reports, 12*, 271–283.

Webster-Stratton, C. H., & Reid, J. (2012). T*ailoring the incredible years: Parent, teacher, and child interventions for young children with ADHD*. http://67.199.123.90/Library/items/Tailoring-the-incredible-years-parent-teacher-child-ADHD-chapter-2014.pdf

Chapter 14
Family Interventions

Roberto Alves Banaco and **Inaldo J. da Silva Júnior**

A frequent complaint observed in psychology clinics applied to problems observed in childhood and adolescence is that formulated by parents: "there was no school for us to learn how to raise our children" (Kazdin & Rotella, 2008; Latham, 1996). For this reason, it is recommended and desirable that the child therapist conduct orientation sessions for parents and other people who live directly with the child.

This recommendation is derived from the observation that, even making use of intervention and producing changes in the child's behavioral repertoire in the therapeutic context, generalization of behavior does not always occur in other environments, such as home and school. The recommendation is to allow parents to identify their own behaviors that may sometimes be producing and/or maintaining the problems they complain about. According to Marinotti (2012), parental guidance is an integral part of the clinical process with the child; however, this guidance may not be enough to achieve the desired changes. In these cases, an alternative to be considered, based on the analysis of the data obtained and the therapist's understanding of the case, is family therapy.

This chapter aims to present family therapy as a resource that can be further explored by behavior analysts and suggests in which context to make use of this model of intervention. Furthermore, it describes some possibilities of therapeutic conduction and lists variables, with the intention that the therapist be sensitive to them, in order to guide the clinical management. We will discuss this theme from the perspective of behavior analysis and contributions of the structural family therapy approach, proposed by the psychiatrist and family therapist Salvador Minuchin. It is worth mentioning that this is not the only model proposed to work with families

R. A. Banaco
Paradigma - Center for Behavioral Sciences and Technology, São Paulo, Brazil
e-mail: roberto@paradigmaac.org

I. J. da Silva Júnior (✉)
Private Practice, São Paulo, Brazil

and that one of the expectations with this text is to stimulate the reader's interest for contents related to family therapy.

The Family and Family Therapy

The importance of intervening in family relationships lies in the fact that the family is the child's first social environment. It is in this environment that the child learns the first and most varied behavioral repertoires. It is also in this environment that their first experiences of subjectivity usually begin to appear. Some examples of basic behaviors that will be necessary for other more complex behaviors are imitate; identify and name the stimuli around them; receive and show affection; take care of themselves (both body and things); develop a sense of collectivity; identify hierarchy and social roles; develop social skills and competencies; identify, name, and deal with emotions and sensations (both their own and others); perceive themselves; and experience the *self*, among others. All these behaviors originate in the social environment surrounding the child. In general, this happens in the family context. It is important, therefore, the way in which family members establish relationships among themselves, because this will influence how each one behaves within the family system and the child's behavior before the world.

Definitions of what a family would be are usually rare, perhaps because the plurality of possible conformations is very vast, often not finding a common link that can be extracted from the essence of the concept "family."

Minuchin et al. (2008) provide the following definition for family:

> A family is a group of people, connected by emotion and/or blood, who have lived long enough to have developed patterns of interaction and stories that justify and explain those patterns of interaction. In their patterned interactions with each other, family members construct each other. This complementary construction in the family web of transactions is both good news and bad news (p. 52).

This definition seemed quite comprehensive to us and can be considered a starting point to address what kind of relationships should be contemplated in a therapeutic family relationship. In this way, we are not referring to a specific model of formation of the family structure but to the social function of the existing relations between the members of a particular group, which is conventionally called family.

Another important aspect for the development of therapeutic work is to take into account the formulation of the analysis of behavior on the development of the repertoire of each individual inserted in social relationships – in this case, in family relationships. As in other interactions with the environment, the behavior of the participant in the family group is motivated by his biological needs for survival – and later, for reproduction – and modeled by his consequences, strengthening or weakening classes of responses. Thus, the family group can determine the variability or restriction of the behavioral repertoire of its members. For this reason, describing, organizing, and intervening in the relationships established among the group members may indicate changes that provide a harmonious and healthy scenario.

It is expected that families experience some situations such as the formation of a new couple; the conception of a baby; the presence of a small child; the entry of children at school age, adolescence, or adulthood; the illness of a member; the death of one of the members; the loss of a job; retirement; the breakup of a marital relationship; the adoption of a child; and the union of partners with children, among others. These experiences are an opportunity to develop new repertoires, but alter previously established relationships, occurring gains and losses for each individual. Because of this, there is a process of adaptation to the new reality, which, depending on the developments, may expand healthy behaviors or show sick relationships.

It is through the process of family therapy that the psychologist can observe and act when events are occurring, when the individual repertoires of members of the family group do not reach the necessary adaptation, without creating an aversive social environment. Another particularity of this model of assistance is the opportunity to change the focus of the problem which is normally attributed to a single individual and to start working with the general functioning of the family, emphasizing the relationships established between its members. To this end, the behavior analyst should pay attention to how the tasks characteristically assigned to the mother, father, husband, wife, child, and sibling, among others, are performed and how relationships are established between these performances.

The theoretical foundation seeks to understand how relationships between family group members are established and the possible interlocking contingencies (Glenn, 1986), in which, as described by Naves and Vasconcelos (2008), the behavior of an individual becomes an occasion or consequence for the behavior of another individual from the same social group. This conception originated in Skinner's (1953/1985) proposition on social behavior, which defines it as a behavior that takes place in the relationship of one person with another or of two or more people in joint relation with the physical environment. One of the advantages of this type of behavior is that all those involved in the social relationship produce a result that would not be produced if the individual contingencies were not interlocking in that way.

A consequence of this proposition is that when we observe a relationship in which someone obtains advantages and another loses them, we will be identifying a bad social relationship, which tends to disintegrate, for example, a man who wants to buy a new car for himself and makes the family save, claiming lack of financial resources is the only one to obtain advantage. This is the keynote of family therapy: identify common goals, in which everyone remains satisfied by being together and locate in which types of relationships this "value" is not happening.

Guidelines for the Therapist

The following are suggestions to the work of the family therapist. Probably some of them will be obvious to some readers, but it is worth remembering them. The physical environment of the therapy should have enough space to accommodate the family comfortably, considering the number of seats, lighting, and air circulation. It is interesting for the therapist to have accessible tissue, water, graphic materials, toys, and games, and it is important, in some cases, to have enough space so that people cannot reach each other when accommodated.

The therapist can determine the length of the session, but the literature recommends that in group therapy, having or not a family configuration, the sessions last between 90 and 120 min. The presence of a therapist is indicated in family groups with more than three members, and the supervision of beginning therapists is fundamental.

The therapist needs to consider that his life and professional experiences, personal values, and theoretical knowledge create a bias in his analysis, which may bias his judgment toward family members who live similar contingencies to his own (Banaco, 2008). For example, a therapist who is a father and contributes significantly to his own household finances may empathize more easily with the complaints of a mother who is the breadwinner. On the other hand, a therapist who has much of his or her needs met by funding from other family members may more easily understand the entitlement claims of a child who is being supported by siblings.

Thus, it is important that both a therapist who attends a family alone and the co-therapists who attend together are always willing to revise their interpretations about the family dynamics. The therapist's self-knowledge and self-observation are required to facilitate the identification of the effects that the speeches and actions of the members of the family group have on him/herself. Furthermore, they help him to identify if, when allying himself to one of the members or to a family subsystem, his conduct is guided by a clinical rationale or if he is allying himself to this person for sharing or even for disagreeing with the values that are being imposed to whom he has allied himself.

Descriptions of what is observed by the behavior analyst should be free of prior moral judgments. They should also show the antecedents and consequences produced by certain responses. The purpose of this procedure is to help family members improve their repertoire of identifying and expressing emotions and thoughts, resolving conflicts, making requests, and identifying the variables that control their responses.

In the sessions, the therapist should ideally focus on the interactions among family members rather than on the interaction with each member. In this way, he can witness how the members relate to each other and help improve interpersonal skills. Another therapeutic task is to identify the target behaviors when they occur in the session so that they can be consequenced as close as possible to their emission. For example, during a family session situation report, the daughter will tell the parents directly how she feels (instead of telling the therapist in front of the parents). Thus, she will emit in therapeutic session the class of responses that is intended to be carried out of the session. At that point, notation of the change that has occurred can be made by the psychologist, which can have a reinforcing effect on this interlocking.

The content of the verbal discourse is adjacent and assists in understanding the case. It is the observation of the interactions between the members of the family group that will be most important. The therapist must be attentive to how the report occurs, the context in which it is presented, the emotional expression of the speaker and listeners, the interactions originated from what was said, and the identification of what is being said beyond the words – for example, with autoclips such as voice intonation, speed, metaphors used, etc., which significantly extend the understanding of the family functioning. This observation helps the therapist to define the therapeutic objectives and identify the interventions to be performed.

It is essential to adapt the interventions and the way of interacting according to the family members, respecting their moral, ethical, and religious values. With children, it is appropriate to stoop down when interacting with them; be succinct, clear, and specific in the verbal account; use playful resources; and carry out interventions with the concrete use of language. Intervention techniques should be subordinate – never sovereign – to the formulation and reformulation of the case and the contingencies present in the session. Therefore, therapists should have in their repertoires the domain of quite diversified techniques for the most different purposes.

In addition, very specific issues concerning the couple's relationship (e.g., sexual life or the intimacy of one of the members of the couple) should be addressed separately from the children's problems, just as, depending on the age and education of the children, issues of their intimacy should be addressed separately from those of their parents. For the family session, issues that affect everyone's contingencies should be reserved.

And, finally, it is recommended to observe, encourage, and allow family members to seek alternatives to deal with a problematic situation, always having in mind, as a guiding sense, the objective of the group. On the other hand, the behavior of the psychologist to list several solutions for a situation may be considered a conduct of little therapeutic effect, because they sound like recommendations. Rodrigues et al. (2014) cite studies by authors from different psychological approaches who found evidence that the therapist's directivity is a determinant of the client's resistance and understand it as an interactional phenomenon, i.e., it may occur according to the style of the therapist's interventions.

Suggestions for Conducting the Process

Based on the data obtained in the initial sessions, the therapist will perform the case formulation that is composed of (a) the identification of the current variables and those related to the history of the family or individuals that maintain the problem behavior, (b) the identification and definition of the classes of behaviors that should be reduced and those that should be expanded, (c) the survey of the interventions that will possibly be used for each of the purposes, (d) the composition of the therapeutic goals defined with the family, and (d) the constant re-evaluation of the psychotherapeutic process with the subsequent reformulation of the clinical case, given that behavior is a process in constant development; or, in other words, the formulation of the case is fluid and needs to be revised during therapy as new data are obtained; otherwise, there is the risk of the professional becoming insensitive to new contingencies that life or the therapy itself have modified.

In order to verify how the family members interact, it is advisable to conduct some sessions without making explicit which behaviors are expected from the participants when expressing their emotions, complaints, and point of view. After defining the objectives and target behaviors of each family member – and of the dyad or triad of therapists – they can be asked to express themselves verbally, attending to certain recommendations (e.g., expressing without judgment, aggressions, ironies, and threats) in order to model some behaviors of affect expression in session.

Minuchin et al. (2008) propose a four-step map to assist the therapist in formulating the case and promoting knowledge of family relationships for its members. Table 14.1 presents the original version and a proposed adaptation to the analytic-behavioral terminology.

Table 14.1 Adaptation of Minuchin, Lee, and Simon's (2008) four-step map summary

	First step	Second step	Third step	Fourth step
Terms of structural family therapy	Decentralize the presenting problem and the symptom carrier	Explore family patterns that may be maintaining the presenting problem	Explore what key family members bring from the past that still influences the present	Redefine the problem and explore options
Proposed adaptation to terms of analytic-behavioral therapy	Expand the unit of analysis. Instead of focusing on the problem situation or on a member, collect data on the family relationships established	To identify, with the family members and through clinical observation, the variables of which the behavior is a function and that may contribute to the maintenance of a problematic repertoire for the family relationship	Seek to understand, principally, how ontogeny and culture may have favored the installation of rules and self-rules and possibly left the individual insensitive to current contingencies. Identify values in broad classes of responses Identify unreported gains for the complaint-behavior in all involved in the episode analyzed	Based on the data obtained and on the functional analysis of family relationships, define which are the behaviors for improvement and the interventions that may be appropriate to the case Identify the "triggers" that can lead to a cascade of behaviors by family members in ways that lead to family distress

During the psychotherapeutic process, the therapist will have the opportunity to identify the classes of responses related to the parental, conjugal, fraternal, filial, and individuality repertoires. The objective is to understand how they are exercised and interact among themselves, verifying if there are conflicts between the roles played, alliances, or subgroups, helping the members of the family group to perceive themselves as a whole, establishing the responsibility of each one, given that each one is context for the response of the other.

The behavior analyst has at his disposal a theoretical and technological framework that supports his practice and, when used, contributes to the well-being of individuals living in groups. The professional can make use of this technology when the work is directed at the family. Some general possibilities of interventions are presented below.

The functional hypothesis established in the formulation of the case is the instrument used by the behavior analyst to diagnose and assess the therapeutic process, being the starting point for the planning and monitoring of interventions (Nery & Fonseca, 2018). If well used, it can also be an instrument that contributes to self-knowledge, to the expansion of the repertoire, and to the occurrence of changes in the repertoires of each participant in family therapy.

The therapist(s) can prepare the family for the use of contingency analysis, helping everyone to make the observation of chained events in which each one of them (the family members) has a participation in the problematic episode. This can be done, initially, through examples extracted from the verbal report of the family members, but preferably should be pointed out in the events that occur in session. Later, with the elaboration of functional analyses through the participation of family members in small behavioral changes, the therapist helps the members of the family group to observe and have control over their interactions.

To increase the likelihood of success in interventions, it is recommended that the therapist(s) share the knowledge produced by behavioral psychology with the family. Latham (1996) lists the following principles: (a) behavior is better modeled by positive consequences than by negative consequences; (b) one can only know whether behavior was punished or reinforced by the course of behavior in the future; (c) behavior is largely a product of the immediate environment; and (d) behavior is modeled by consequences. Guided by these principles, the therapist may present the concepts of reinforcement and punishment, extinction, contiguity and contingency, reinforcement schemes, modeling, shaping, establishing operations, arbitrary and natural reinforcers, and aversive control, among others. It is recommended that professionals, when transmitting these concepts, whenever possible, use information obtained through the report of the members of the family group and the events observed during the session.

The principles of behavior analysis that are taught to the family will of course be used by the therapist in session for interventions. For example, as proposed by Delitti and Derdyk (2012), modeling and instruction can be used by the clinician in a planned manner to teach a specific repertoire during the therapy session. Delitti and Derdyk report that: "From behavioral modeling and rehearsals, it is possible to install or change many behaviors, from the behavior of observing oneself and others, analyzing and describing contingencies, social skills, empathy, communication, self-disclosure, coping, etc." (Delitti & Derdyk, 2012, p. 265). The authors emphasize that, for the modeling strategy to be effective, it is necessary to describe the problem situation, decompose the behavioral sequence, give instructions or performance model, rehearse, hint about the performance, program generalization, and assess the performance in the natural situation.

The therapist, when reporting his sensations, emotions, and thoughts as a result of a situation observed in session, can also serve as a model for the family members of how to express verbally their limits and inconveniences in an adequate manner. Depending on the circumstance, by making public the effect that the family members' responses have on him, it is possible to use this data to help model better responses and the perception of their effect on the listener.

Another procedure that aids the installation and strengthening of certain client responses is modeling: the precursor responses of the desirable response are initially reinforced, and as they are established, reinforcement gradually moves to new responses hierarchically closer to the target response (Del Prette & García, 2007, p.185).

A basic recommendation that should start the whole therapeutic process is the use of positive reinforcement rather than coercive control because it produces the strengthening of affective interactions and improves life values and the behavioral repertoire of the people involved. Emphasizing the bond between parents and children, as stated by Sidman (1989/2009), is a way to help children to have a productive and happy life, without feeling they need to do something special to get love and protection. In addition, it is to provide an environment in which they feel safe and that, even if they do something wrong, they still know they will have protection and affection.

As mentioned elsewhere in this text, the therapist must privilege interventions related to the events that occur in session. Yalom and Leszcz (2006) understands that for this to occur, the therapist needs to help the group to get involved in the here-and-now experience and help them to understand the process of the experience, that is, to get in touch with the contingencies present in the interaction. The ability to focus on the present moment allows the members of the family group to identify more easily the triggers of their good and bad behaviors, as well as their tendencies to respond to the issues of the family relationship. They can then make more conscious choices about how to act.

In order to achieve these objectives, it is necessary to be aware of what is happening in the present moment; observe and, when appropriate, describe the internal and external events in face of the situations experienced in session by the family members and therapists; and identify and consequentize the clinically relevant behaviors, which are already described in the case formulation. Therapists who adhere to the therapeutic process known as FAP (functional analytic psychotherapy) describe these behaviors as clinically relevant behaviors (clinical relevant behaviors – CRBs). In these processes, therapists should recognize functional parallels between behaviors presented in session and those that occur in clients' lives outside the office, enhance behaviors of vulnerability, and use the therapeutic relationship as a model of interaction for family members. Hoekstra and Tsai (2010) state that FAP provides a theoretical framework and format for behavior analysts who work with groups and focus on improving interpersonal relationships.

It is also possible to use therapeutic resources described by ACT (acceptance and commitment therapy) to help the family identify and behave toward their values. Brandão (2008) understands that elucidating the clients' values and commitments to act according to the established goals is a didactic way to start the sessions. Having a family's values clear helps therapists to define broad classes of target responses to which they can direct the behavioral repertoires to be installed in each family member. The model proposed by ACT can help the therapist, through relational *frame* theory (RFT), to understand and reveal the frames established in the family relationship. In other words, succinctly, it reveals how excessive verbal control and arbitrarily established relationships may influence the maintenance of a limited repertoire that is not very flexible and insensitive to reinforcing contingencies.

It is worth emphasizing that what has been discussed so far will only make sense if professionals and members of the family group, when evaluating the results obtained, notice changes that promote improvement in family interactions beyond the clinic. Therefore, the planning of generalization of the behaviors worked on in the clinical context must be considered by the therapist whenever he elaborates his intervention plan.

Final Considerations

This chapter was aimed at identifying some situations that can produce changes in family relationships, which in turn can considerably affect the behavior of children. Parental guidance skills are sufficient to conduct several therapeutic processes for children, but sometimes the origin of the problems faced and experienced by children is found in the family relationships themselves. It is up to the therapist to identify if and when guidance will be sufficient and when a more robust therapeutic process should be conducted to solve the problems brought to the clinic.

Changes in structural living conditions – such as the entrance and/or exit of someone in the family life – usually produce great influence on the child's social relations, demanding that the adaptation process be conducted in a safe and coherent way. The process should be conducted so that everyone in the family can benefit from the changes pursued by the indications of the behavioral formulation. The therapist must consider the behavior of each family member as the social context in which the behavior of the other family component occurs, distributing to all the problem and the weight of the intervention and of the change. The family becomes "having a problem" and not just "having a child who was considered problematic."

The proposals of adaptation described by Minuchin et al. (2008) in analytic-behavioral terms were presented, so as to be followed by the therapist as a set of rules. They are guidelines for a good family service, and the reader can find in the literature cited below other works that are of aid to the conduction of a complex process, such as the therapy of the "family" group. Because it is complex, the work in co-therapy is indicated, and the supervision of the case receives special attention, so that the therapist(s) do not incur in common and probable mistakes, specially empathizing with one or part of the family members.

The great advantage of therapy conducted this way is that the processes to be worked on will be manifested under the eye and technique of the therapist(s). In short, parents can have a school to learn how to develop their children's behaviors.

References

Banaco, R. A. (2008). A terapia analítico-comportamental em um grupo especial: A terapia de famílias. In M. Delitti & P. Derdyk (Eds.), *Terapia Analítico-Comportamental em Grupo* (pp. 195–212). ESETec Editores Associados.

Brandão, M. Z. S. (2008). Esquiva experiencial do cliente no grupo terapêutico e promoção de aceitação emocional. In: Delitti, M., Derdyk, P. *Terapia Analítico-Comportamental em Grupo*. (pp. 61-91). ESETec Editores Associados.

Del Prette, G., & García, R. M. (2007). Técnicas comportamentais: possibilidades e vantagens no atendimento em ambiente extraconsultório. In D. R. Zamignani, R. Kovac, & J. S. Vermes (Eds.), *A clínica de portas abertas: experiências e fundamentação do acompanhamento terapêutico e da prática clínica em ambiente extraconsultório* (pp. 183–200). ESETec Editores Associados e Paradigma – Núcleo de Análise do Comportamento.

Delitti, M., & Derdyk, P. (2012). O trabalho da análise do comportamento com grupos: possibilidades de aplicação a casais e família. In N. B. Borges & F. A. Cassas (Eds.), *Clínica Analítico-Comportamental: aspectos teóricos e práticos* (pp. 259–269). ArtMed.

Glenn, S. S. (1986). Metacontingencies in Walden two. *Behavior Analysis and Social Action, 5*, 2–8.

Hoekstra, R., & Tsai, M. (2010). FAP for interpersonal process groups. In J. W. Kanter, M. Tsai, & R. J. Kohlenberg (Eds.), (pp. 247–260). Springer.

Kazdin, A. E., & Rotella, C. (2008). *The Kazdin method for parenting the defiant child: With no pills, no therapy, no contest of wills*. Mariner Books.

Latham, G. I. (1996). The making of a stable family. In J. R. Cautela & W. Ishaq (Eds.), *Contemporary issues in behavior therapy*. Plenum Press.

Marinotti, M. (2012). A importância da participação da família na clínica analítico-comportamental infantil. In N. B. Borges & F. A. Cassas (Eds.), *Clínica Analítico-Comportamental: aspectos teóricos e práticos* (pp. 251–258). Artmed.

Minuchin, S., Lee, W., & Simon, G. M. (2008). *Dominando a terapia familiar (tradução Gisele Klein)* (2nd ed.). Artmed.

Naves, A. R. C. X., & Vasconcelos, l. A. (2008). O estudo da família: contingências e metacontingências. *Revista Brasileira de Análise do Comportamento/Brazilian Journal of Behavior Analysis, 4*(1), 13–25.

Nery, L. B., & Fonseca, F. N. (2018). Análises funcionais moleculares e molares: um passo a passo. In A. K. C. R. De Farias, F. N. Fonseca, & L. B. Nery (Eds.), *Teoria e formulação de casos em análise comportamental clínica* (pp. 22–54). Artmed.

Rodrigues, B. D., Lima, C. F., Malavazzi, D. M., Zamignani, D. R., Filho, E. S., Del Prette, G., Mazer, M., Zuccolo, P. F., Banaco, R. A., Almeida, T. A. C., & Mangabeira, V. (2014). Efeitos de intervenções reflexivas sobre o repertório do cliente no processo terapêutico analítico-comportamental. In D. R. Zamignani & S. B. Meyer (Eds.), *A pesquisa de processo em psicoterapia: estudos a partir do instrumento SiMCCIT – Sistema Multidimensional para a Categorização de Comportamento na Interação Terapêutica* (Vol. 2, 1st ed., pp. 145–165). Paradigma Núcleo de Análise do Comportamento.

Sidman, M. (2009). *Coerção e suas implicações* (trad. M. M. Andery, T. M. Sério). Editoria Livro Pleno. (Trabalho original publicado em 1989).

Skinner, B. F. (1953/1985). In J. C. Todorov & R. Azzi (Eds.), *Ciência e comportamento humano* (6th ed.).

Yalom, I. D. & Leszcz, M. (2006). *Psicoterapia de grupo: teria e prática*. (trad. R. C. Costa). 5th ed. Artmed.

Suggested Readings

Kohlenberg, R. J., & Tsai, M. (1991). Functional analytic psychotherapy: Creating intense and curative therapeutic relationships. *Plenum Press.* https://doi.org/10.1007/978-0-387-70855-3

Martins Jade, C. T. Lustosa Leite, Felipe, Metacontingências e Macrocontingências: Revisão de pesquisas experimentais brasileiras. Acta Comportamentalia: Revista Latina de Análisis de Comportamiento 2016, 24 (dez. – jan.,2017) http://www.redalyc.org/articulo.oa?id=274548797005

Minuchin, S., & Fishman, H. C. (1990). *Técnicas de terapia familiar* (tradução Kinsh, C., & Maia, M. E. F. R.). Artmed.

Chapter 15
Therapeutic Discharge as an Outcome of Clinical Behavior Analysis for Children: Criteria and Process

Clarissa Moreira Pereira and Daniel Del Rey

What Is Therapeutic Discharge?

For didactic purposes, we will call "therapeutic discharge" the process of closing the psychological sessions due to the conclusion of the behavioral goals proposed at the beginning of the therapy and the absence of new relevant goals throughout the process. Although extremely important, this topic has been little addressed in the literature (Patterson et al., 2009). Theoretically, therapeutic discharge with children is indicated by the professional and discussed with the family, seeking mutual agreement.

It is important to specify the term "discharge," because many times the process can be interrupted or terminated, without necessarily having achieved the proposed objectives. In the case of interventions with children, in general, the decision for early termination is made by the family and can be related to several issues, such as (a) financial or logistical difficulties, (b) disagreement with the therapist, (c) resistance of the child with the therapist and/or psychotherapy, (d) difficulties in implementing the proposed strategies, and (e) using the time for other activities considered more urgent by the family, such as academic support. In other situations, the therapist may choose to terminate the process early, usually for lack of competence with some particular topic or repertoire (in these cases, the client is referred to another professional). None of these options could be termed "discharge" since the reasons for discontinuing the process are unrelated to the goals established for the intervention.

Thus, a therapeutic discharge process can only be well conducted if, throughout the process, clinical goals have been well defined and somehow well followed up. If measurement units could be used to follow their evolution, so much the better.

C. M. Pereira (✉) · D. D. Rey
Paradigma - Center for Behavioral Sciences and Technology, São Paulo, SP, Brazil

Based on the definition presented above, this chapter aims to discuss how to (a) assess the demand that brings a child to therapy (initial assessment or diagnosis), (b) outline the therapeutic goals (behavioral intervention) based on the complaint and the initial assessment, (c) assess whether the goals were met throughout the process, and (d) proceed to therapeutic discharge taking into account not only whether the child acquired important socioemotional repertoires for the prevention of future problems and a healthy development but also the generalization of these repertoires to the natural environment (Müller & Quaschner, 2001).

Specificities in the Therapeutic Process with Children

Reflecting on the therapeutic discharge process with children may be more complex than with adult clients. The first point of this complexity is due to the variety of relevant agendas that permeate children's lives, as well as the speed with which new topics relevant to the therapeutic process arise during this stage of life, changing the direction of the original intervention.

A second issue concerns the fact that the work with children is not restricted to contact with them, often involving the family, the school, and other professionals who make up the interdisciplinary team or who work together with the child, such as speech therapists, neurologists or psychiatrists, private teachers, etc. Differently from therapy with adults, the initiative to seek psychological assistance and the identification of their goals are rarely taken by the children themselves. Children rarely request psychotherapy and describe their goals; most of the time it is the family who decides to start the process, by their own initiative or through guidance from the school or other professionals. During the therapeutic process, often the psychologist himself formulates goals from observation and reports of children, but this ends up adding to the demands of the family or those who made the referral.

Thus, the discharge process involves several demands, not only those brought initially, increasing the number of relevant variables to be observed throughout the intervention. Some of these specificities will be briefly addressed here.

Initial Assessment

First, it is worth noting that when talking about diagnosis or behavioral assessment, the behavior analyst should take into account the procedural nature of the behavior. In other words, there is no separation between assessment and intervention; at different times, they overlap (Vermes, 2012). Therefore, while conducting interviews, observation, and activities with the child and his family, the therapist should consider the possibility of changes in the variables relevant to the observed behavior and, thus, a possible behavioral change already at that moment.

Del Prette et al. (2005) analyzed 20 case studies published in Brazil with children as the focus of the interventions. The work aimed to analyze the evaluation methods used in the studies that would attest their internal validity. According to the authors, the procedures most commonly cited in the literature as relevant to the initial assessment process are (a) interview with parents, (b) interview with the child, (c) interview with other significant others, (d) medical assessment, (e) records (by parents, professionals, or the child itself), (f) direct observation, and (g) use of tests. The use of different procedures would increase the internal validity of the study, since it would allow a better functional analysis of the case and a greater chance of success of the proposed treatment. In the survey carried out, the initial interview with parents and direct observation of the children's behavior were the most used procedures. At the end of the intervention, most of the studies did not refer to repeating the initial measures, only performing a new observation of the child's behavior. As discussed by the authors, despite the difficulties in carrying out a systematic and exhaustive evaluation of case studies, it is extremely important to have the most accurate evaluation possible of the intervention, which, unfortunately, still does not occur in the national production of behavior analysis.

Another point discussed in the study relates the diversity of demands to the diversity of assessment strategies used, since each procedure applies better to specific issues. The procedures will be discussed in some detail, as it is considered that without a good initial assessment, it is not possible to define clear criteria for therapeutic discharge.

Interview with Parents or Caregivers

Once the parents arrive for the initial interview, the therapist should seek the reasons why they were sought. It is interesting to identify, at this moment, if the reasons mentioned by the different caregivers are similar. The initial interviews can even be conducted separately with each of them (e.g., Fonseca & Pacheco, 2010).

It is important to seek information to evaluate factors that may be contributing to the problem and also to identify well-developed repertoires of the child that may facilitate improvements. The therapist should investigate the genetic history of the child and family members, the child's developmental history from gestation to birth and early childhood, health history and medical complaints, attachment history and parental separation (long trips, separation/divorce between parents), the relationship between parents and between parents and child, the environment in which the child lives, the family constitution, relationships, family history (cultural, religious, and values), school/academic complaints or issues, and social complaints (Adler-Tapia, 2012).

After collecting life history data, they proceed to the analysis of the present moment. Questions about the child's routine are extremely important and, when answered separately by the different caregivers, may provide complementary information. The questions should be asked in order to seek possible functional relationships between the behavior and environment variables. Parents are asked about when the behavior occurs, what it looks like, in the presence of which people it occurs more often, and what happens in the situation after the behavior occurs, among others.

It is also of utmost importance that the therapist investigates the possibility of occurrence of episodes of abuse or violence, self-harm or suicide attempts, and substance use by family members, given the impact that such factors may have on the child's behavior and, therefore, on the therapeutic complaint (Patterson et al., 2009).

Some standardized instruments can be applied to parents and caregivers to obtain the information initially collected, such as anamnesis questionnaires, inventories on behavior (*Child Behavior Checklist*, by Bordin et al., 1995, for example), or *checklist* for some specific disorders (SNAP-IV scale to assess ADHD, for example – Mattos et al., 2006).

Interview and Observation with the Child

The initial interview with the child meets two objectives simultaneously: to begin to structure the therapeutic relationship and collect information. In this chapter, we will focus on the second part. When we interview children, we have a wide range of singularities that depend on variables such as age group, repertoire, medical diagnosis, motivation to collaborate, and socioeconomic level, among others. This creates limitations and requires technical adaptations. For example, an older child, motivated to collaborate and with a good verbal repertoire, may provide several pieces of information by means of a report. A younger child, on the other hand, who is upset because he or she is with a stranger or has some invasive syndrome, for example, will hardly collaborate verbally. Due to these different situations, in some more favorable conditions, the child's verbal report may prove to be a good source of relevant data for the analysis process. However, since all data collection resources have limitations, it will always be necessary for the therapist to use various resources to obtain information to enrich the analysis, including direct observation of behavior.

Observation of the child's behavior can be done both in the office and in the natural environment (at home or at school, for example). When done in the office, the therapist can use some resources to evoke behavior and observe possible variables relevant to it. Games, jokes, or fantasies can fulfill this function. The topography of relevant behaviors may be different from that which occurs outside the session, but maintaining, however, functional similarities that allow the therapist direct access to classes of relevant behaviors (Moreira & Oshiro, 2017).

When observation is performed in the natural environment, in addition to being able to conduct pre-defined structured evaluations according to specific objectives, the therapist has access to data on how the child relates to his/her physical and social environment in loco, with less external interference. Although the very presence of the observer is a variable that may contaminate the observation, it is possible to obtain valuable information on the environmental organization, routine, social environment, and aspects of interpersonal relationships of the environment to be analyzed with less distortion than occurs when verbal reporting is used.

Interview with Significant Others

Interviews with significant others have the same objectives as the interview with parents or caregivers, that is, to collect data on target behaviors (and their functional relationships) and competencies that may help the process, but in other contexts. It is very common for teachers, babysitters, drivers, other staff, and other family members to see relevant behaviors that parents do not see. This can occur both because of differences in the activities performed and repertoires involved in each of the different environments and the evocative function of each of these people. Regardless of the reason, the analysis becomes more complete with more sources of information. For example, the description of a child who is able to be extremely collaborative with teachers and peers, but refuses to obey simple parental rules, already adds very useful information to the analysis.

Proposal and Implementation of the Intervention

Once the initial analysis is complete, the relevant behaviors are divided into two broad categories: (a) classes of responses to be installed/strengthened and (b) classes of responses to be weakened. The classes of responses to be installed or strengthened in general are repertoires linked to academic, playful, and interpersonal activities. These responses may already be present in children's repertoires and appear with low frequency (requiring strengthening) or have not been taught (still needing to be installed). In general, new skills not present in children's repertoires are installed by shaping or instruction. The choice of each of these strategies is determined by the child's age group, level of impairment, previous competence, and repertoire to be taught. For these strategies to work, it is essential that the clinician and the people who will intervene have powerful reinforcers available, using them contingently to the new responses throughout the process.

The responses that need to be weakened refer to behaviors that are, in some way, causing problems for the child or those around him. In general, these responses are related to tantrums, aggression, self-injury, repetitive behaviors, or excessive behaviors that compete with other important activities. These are responses that, although maintained by negative or positive reinforcement, bring other harmful consequences, even in the medium or long term. The most frequently used strategy to weaken responses is differential reinforcement, in which the response that needs to decrease in frequency will not be reinforced or will be reinforced at a lower intensity than other competing responses, opposite or alternative to the original. Differential reinforcement turns out to be a better alternative than punishing or simply not reinforcing that response (behavioral extinction), since it avoids or minimizes side effects such as counter-control or emotional responses, in addition to installing more functional repertoires under the control of more appropriate stimuli.

In addition to the intervention with the child, it is essential that the therapist conducts counseling sessions with parents and people relevant to the child, such as teachers, babysitters, or other relatives. This guidance seeks to make people related to the target behaviors change their attitudes, modifying the children's environment in order to change their behaviors. Therapeutic discharge will probably not occur in situations where the only new variable is the therapist's presence. It is necessary that the child's social environment also changes, new patterns having been selected.

Assessment of the Changes that Occurred in Therapy

Both in the direct work with children and in parental guidance, the assessment of the evolution of target behaviors is carried out continuously, i.e., throughout the intervention process. The data arising from a continuous evaluation process allow for the identification of the following: (1) procedures, their effectiveness and possible reformulation of the same; (2) engagement of the family, school, and significant others with the proposed analysis and intervention; if necessary, such data will serve as an element for analysis of the difficulties encountered in the implementation of the proposals and for possible adjustments; and (3) identification of the results themselves in relation to the objectives established.

When a family seeks therapy for their child, the goal will invariably be to produce improvement in the quality of life of the child and the family. Improvement is evaluated in a qualitative way, and, for this reason, it may incur in judgment errors due to biases that hinder the evaluation. Kazdin (2000) lists some of these biases that may compromise the evaluation of the therapeutic process: (a) connections between events are made from stereotypes or expected relations, (b) evaluations are made about a case from another similar one, (c) first impressions are used for some evaluations, (d) hypotheses are formulated from the therapist's personal beliefs, and (e) correlations are observed and causes are inferred from there, without direct testing.

Because of this problem, the author stresses the importance of more precise tools for the evaluation of the gains from the therapy, which is often only possible in the case of a clinical experimental research. In any case, some points raised by him deserve attention, even if they are difficult to implement in office practice. One of them would be the continuous evaluation of the problem behavior, not only before and after the intervention but also during it. Another point would be the formulation of an intervention design, in which the moment when the intervention procedure is implemented and changes in behavior can be observed and recorded is clearly marked.

A clinical practice that has contributed to the increased reliability of therapy outcomes is case formulation.

> A case formulation in psychotherapy is a hypothesis about the causes, precipitants, and sustaining influences of a person's psychological, interpersonal, and behavioral problems. A case formulation helps to organize information about a person [...]. Ideally, it contains structures that allow the therapist to understand [...] and categorize important classes of information within a sufficiently comprehensive view of the patient. A case formulation also serves as a treatment guide and as a marker of change (Eells, 2007, p. 4).

By listing the components of the functional analysis, separating and sequencing them in a narrative or schematic structure, and reformulating them as the treatment proceeds, the therapist can reduce the number of inferences he needs to make about the case. This assessment is extremely relevant, since only after reaching the therapeutic goals is it possible to proceed to discharge.

Maintenance, Generalization, and Relapse Prevention

There are numerous strategies to be implemented aiming at generalizing the changes achieved in therapy, maximizing the probability of the gains being maintained after discharge. One of them is the spacing of the sessions added to a greater focus on parental guidance. Through this strategy, the therapist can fade out the bond and control with the child, while the family gains confidence in managing different situations of conflict/difficulties.

Parental guidance is a prerequisite for intervention with children, since parents will control the main reinforcing contingencies of their children for many years, manipulating the most important reinforcers, describing the first rules, and providing the first role models. If the family and/or caregivers adopt inappropriate practices most of the time, it will make little or no difference a few hours a week in office sessions with the child. Therefore, if we can get parents to understand and follow basic guidelines, the chance that changes will occur throughout the process and continue after the sessions are over increases dramatically. To this end, it is important that the clinician uses strategies beyond verbal instruction, such as shaping observation and description behavior of the child's behavior, problem-solving and decision-making training for problem situations that may arise in the daily life with the child, and modeling the ability to functionally analyze behavior, among others (Marinotti, 2012).

Another relevant aspect still in relation to parental guidance is the outsourcing that has been done in relation to the upbringing of children. Whether due to overwork and other activities or the difficulty in finding parameters of how to position themselves with their children, parents seem less and less able to clearly set limits to children and teach important life skills. This situation requires care because at the same time that child therapy can empower and call the family to the responsibility of educating, it can also serve the function of delegating these responsibilities to a third party, in this case the therapist.

If this is the case, the discharge process becomes more painful for all and much more difficult to happen, since for the family the situation is comfortable and the maintenance of this bond becomes more important. The emergence of several clinically irrelevant agendas, with the function of maintaining the therapy, can evidence this type of relationship of dependence. It is essential that, in these cases, the family is made aware of its importance for the child's behavior and that guidance is given with the purpose of teaching them positive and propositional parenting skills. It may be interesting to refer parents to a therapeutic group, for example, that serves this purpose.

Another option to ensure the maintenance of gains would be sessions in a natural environment. In these *settings*, the intervener could observe and act on the child's behavior, as well as guide other relevant people in his environment to act in a manner consistent with the principles of the intervention. Since this work helps obtain data in loco, not depending on verbal mediation of behavior, it is easier to understand possible difficulties in generalizing certain behaviors. Situations are not rare where family members or caregivers report acting according to the guidelines, but in practice behave in other ways. The report on their own behavior may be compromised by self-observation difficulties, verbal limitations, or avoidance. Regardless of the reason, direct observation allows both better analysis of target behaviors and a contextualized intervention, facilitating the maintenance of relevant post-intervention changes.

Although much of the focus of behavioral interventions is related to target behaviors related to the main demands, there are a number of other important aspects for discharge and relapse prevention. The reappearance of problem behaviors after the end of therapy can occur for numerous factors, including the following: the intervention was restricted to some instances of relevant response classes, but contingencies maintaining the class continued to operate on other functionally equivalent responses, and original contingencies (prior to the intervention) operate again, either in environments involved in the intervention or in new environments to which the client now has access, among others. Below, we mention some precautions at the end of therapy that reduce the probability of the problem returning.

A first important characteristic to be worked on concerns the clients' overall behavioral variety, despite the attention given to specific complaints. If the therapeutic process can help broaden response topographies, subjects of interest, environments frequented, or forms of interpersonal relationships, the likelihood of maintenance of and access to reinforcing stimuli will be much greater.

Expanding the repertoire of life skills is also extremely important. *Life* skills are the following:

> [...] adaptive and positive behavioral skills that enable individuals to deal effectively with the demands and challenges of everyday life. In particular, life skills are a group of psychosocial competencies and interpersonal skills that help people make informed decisions, solve problems, think critically and creatively, communicate effectively, build healthy relationships, empathize with others, and cope with their lives in a healthy and productive manner. Life skills can be directed toward personal actions or actions in relation to others, as well as actions that modify the surrounding environment to make it conducive to health (World Health Organization, 2003).

Problem-solving, one of the life skills, is another of the fundamental objectives to be worked on in the sessions and should also be in the decision to terminate therapy. If the client has a robust repertoire and is skilled in choosing appropriate responses to each situation, he/she will probably efficiently dodge aversive contingencies, as well as have a more effective approach in the search for relevant reinforcers. Cooper, Heward, and Heron (2013) highlight basic procedures to ensure this repertoire, such as training problem-solving responses in various conditions of different stimuli, as well as various topographies for the same class of responses, ensuring a variety that suits different contexts. Among the classes of relevant responses for problem-solving, we can highlight the following: relating data and deriving conclusions; listing different alternatives for dealing with similar situations; and, when faced with new situations, for which the client does not have responses in his/her repertoire or is prevented from doing so for some reason, issuing responses that may lead to the solution response (preliminary or precursor responses).

The development of self-management or self-control repertoire is another relevant objective of the therapeutic process, either because it is directly related to the problem presented by the client or because it constitutes an essential repertoire to avoid future problems. Behavioral variability and problem-solving skills constitute facilitating conditions for self-management. However, some conditions are fundamental for this to be effectively developed, such as resistance to frustration, efficient control by delayed reinforcers, and behavior maintenance by intermediate reinforcers, since many self-control situations involve conflicts between immediate *versus* delayed consequences, such as immediate positive consequences *versus* delayed aversive conditions (playing with friends and not studying for a test), immediate aversive consequences *versus* delayed positive consequences (depriving oneself of caloric foods aiming at substantial weight loss in the medium term), etc.

Additionally, it is important to consider, at discharge, whether clients are able to conduct functional analyses independently, that is, whether they can identify basic behavioral control variables that act on their behavior or on the behavior of others, an ability that facilitates engagement in self-control or problem-solving responses. Obviously this is a more sophisticated skill that needs to be developed, imposing adaptations according to the client's age group and global repertoire.

Finally, it is important to consider the contingencies in place in the natural environment when deciding the moment of discharge. The therapeutic process is not limited to installing/strengthening or extinguishing/weakening classes of responses but also involves changes in contingencies in order to reduce aversive ones and increase control by positive contingencies. Thus, when considering the closure of the process, it is fundamental that we analyze the contingencies in operation to evaluate the probability of maintenance and generalization of gains resulting from therapy.

Farewell: How to Proceed to Discharge

As described by Vermes (2012), in any therapeutic discharge process, it is necessary to consider that there will be a separation of the child from a person who has probably become important in his/her life. Therefore, some care should be taken. The child cannot identify the interruption of the process as a loss but rather as an achievement. For that, it is important to list with the child which changes occurred throughout the sessions, emphasizing passages and clinically relevant or overcoming moments.

Another important precaution is to make it clear that there is always the possibility of resuming the sessions in the future, either by holding a few sessions to discuss specific issues or by resuming a longer-lasting therapy process, provided there is demand for it. The idea that the end of the sessions is not necessarily a definitive goodbye helps the child to accept the end of the sessions and facilitates possible future contact, since the door has been kept open. It is worth explaining to the child that life has many phases and challenges, and it is not a demerit to ask for help in the future if the situation changes.

Finally, as suggested earlier, appointments should be initially spaced out before full closure, minimizing the impact of the separation. It is common for some clients to feel sad or angry at the end of the process, just as others will feel happy or relieved. These emotional responses carry information not exclusively about the therapeutic relationship but about the therapeutic process as a whole. Many clients would like to use session time for other more pleasurable activities or see therapy as evidence that there is something bad or wrong with them, even if it was an agenda during the sessions.

Some therapists feel comfortable maintaining occasional and sporadic contact with their former clients. Such practice, although optional, can help in this separation process and provide data for follow-up. But it also requires care so that it is not characterized as an informal psychotherapy process or a personal/affectionate relationship between the therapist and his former client. If there is relevant clinical demand in these contacts, the ideal is to make new formal appointments. And if the client-professional relationship has become too intimate, it is recommended that the sessions be referred to a colleague.

Final Considerations

As previously discussed, the therapeutic discharge process is complex and is directly related to a well-done and continuous assessment. It is extremely common for the original agenda to give way to other issues, especially as children acquire increasingly earlier repertoires that were previously restricted to adolescence and adulthood, mainly due to their exposure to multiple contexts (out-of-school activities) and the use of the Internet and social networks. These new guidelines bring great insecurity to families, who seek specialized help to know how to proceed and help children to deal with them.

In addition to directly addressing the initial complaints, it is essential to implement strategies that produce generalized and stable changes over time and across different environments. In addition, training of specific repertoires such as problem-solving and contingency analysis may help to reduce the risk of relapse after the end of the intervention.

Once the therapist has sufficient data regarding relevant behavioral changes and indicators of gain maintenance and relapse prevention, other planned procedures should be put in place to minimize the impacts of separation on the client. As a final step in the process, it is important that the client is able to identify if he needs to resume the process and feels comfortable resuming contact with the professional.

References

Adler-Tapia, R. (2012). *Child psychotherapy: Integrating developmental theory into clinical practice*. Springer.

Bordin, I. A. S., Mari, J. J., & Caeiro, M. F. (1995). Validação da versão brasileira do "Child Behavior Checklist" (CBCL) (Inventário de Comportamentos da Infância e Adolescência): dados preliminares. *Revista da Associação Brasileira de Psiquiatria, 17*(2), 55–66.

Cooper, H., & Heward. (2013). *Applied behavior analysis*. Pearson Education.

Del Prette, G., Silvares, E. F. M., & Meyer, S. B. (2005). Validade interna em 20 estudos de caso comportamentais brasileiros sobre terapia infantil. *Revista Brasileira de Terapia Comportamental e Cognitiva, 7*(1), 93–105.

Eells, T. D. (2007). *Handbook of psychotherapy case formulation*. The Guilford Press.

Fonseca, R. P., & Pacheco, J. T. B. (2010). Análise funcional do comportamento na avaliação e terapia com crianças. *Revista Brasileira de Terapia Comportamental e Cognitiva, 12*(1), 1–19.

Kazdin, A. E. (2000). *Psychotherapy for children and adolescents: Directions for research and practice*. Oxford University Press.

Marinotti, M. (2012). A importância da família na clínica analítico-comportamental infantil, Chap. 25. In N. B. Borges & F. A. Cassas (Eds.), *Clínica analítico-comportamental: aspectos teóricos e práticos* (Vol. 1, pp. 251–258). Artmed.

Mattos, P., Serra-Pinheiro, M. A., Rohde, L. A., & Pinto, D. (2006). Apresentação de uma versão em português para uso no Brasil do instrumento MTA-SNAP-IV de avaliação de sintomas de transtorno do déficit de atenção/hiperatividade e sintomas de transtorno desafiador e de oposição. *Revista de Psiquiatria do Rio Grande do Sul, 28*(3), 290–297.

Moreira, F. R., & Oshiro, C. K. B. (2017). Reflexões sobre terapia analítico-comportamental infantil e psicoterapia analítico-funcional com crianças. *Revista Brasileira de Terapia Comportamental e Cognitiva, 19*(3), 166–184.

Müller, U., & Quaschner, K. (2001). Behaviour therapy, Chap. 6. In H. Remschmidt (Ed.), *Psychotherapy with children and adolescents* (Vol. 1, pp. 98–112). Cambridge University Press.

Organização Mundial da Saúde. (2003). *Skills for health: Skills-based health education including life skills: An important component of a child-friendly/health-promoting school*. World Health Organization.

Patterson, J., Williams, L., Edwards, T. M., Chamow, L., & Grauf-Grounds, C. (2009). *Essencial skills in family therapy: From the first interview to termination* (Rev. ed.). The Gilford Press.

Vermes, J. S. (2012). Clínica analítico-comportamental infantil: a estrutura, Chap. 24. In N. B. Borges & F. A. Cassas (Eds.), *Clínica analítico-comportamental: aspectos teóricos e práticos* (Vol. 1, pp. 214–222). Artmed.

Chapter 16
Ethical Issues in Clinical Behavior Analysis for Children

Lygia T. Durigon and Enzo B. Bissoli

The concept of ethics is traditionally defined as a set of rules of conduct, proposed to a given social group and is often used as a synonym for morality (La Taille, 2006). The origin of the words differs – *ethos* comes from Greek and *mores* from Latin – but both refer to "the field of reflection on the customs of men" (La Taille, 2006, p. 25) or "the customs and practices of the group" (Skinner, 1972, 1976a, b, p.107), which justifies the equivalent use of the terms. Skinner (1972, 1976a, b) uses this convention and does not distinguish moral from ethics throughout his work. His reflections on these concepts appear when he discusses cultural practices that contribute to (or hinder) the evolution of a given culture.

For Skinner (1972, 1976a, b), the evolution of a culture is closely related to the adoption of practices that ensure its survival. However, this does not always occur. Acting under control of what is immediately reinforcing for oneself or for others can generate immediate and, mainly, delayed consequences that conflict with the survival of the culture. Examples of products of contingencies of this type are overpopulation, environmental pollution, decreasing resources, and the risk of nuclear wars (Skinner, 1972, 1976a, b).

Planning for a culture must therefore include establishing contingencies that lead individuals to behave in ways that preserve it. One of the ways the group uses for this is assuming the role of determining what is "good" or "bad" and "right" or "wrong." When this occurs, one enters the field of ethics (Ferreira, 2018). It is through the establishment of contingencies of reinforcement and punishment (Skinner, 1953/2000) that a group of people defines and controls ethical behaviors. What is determined as ethical, however, varies according to the context and the historical moment (Gianfaldoni, 2005).

Just as ethical behaviors are culturally defined, so are ethical guidelines for a particular group (Vandenbergue, 2005). In the context of the psychologist's

---

L. T. Durigon (✉) · E. B. Bissoli
Private Practice, São Paulo, Brazil

professional practice, ethical behaviors are delimited and systematized generally in documents, codes of ethics, or even laws and resolutions. Their formats will depend on the regional and historical contexts in which each group is inserted, and it is always essential that the therapist is aware of them, as well as monitor and participate in their construction, review, and change processes.

In part, how each individual will behave when faced with each ethical recommendation will depend on what was selected in his or her life history (Vandenbergue, 2005). However, in order to *ensure* a standard of conduct or to *hold* the individual *accountable*, coercive contingencies are established to punish behaviors defined as unethical.

Noncompliance with the determinations incurs, on an individual level, inspection by peers, which generally take the name of ethics committees and, when deemed pertinent, penalties to the professional, which may be warnings, fines, public censure, suspension, or even revocation of professional practice. The specificity of the documents as well as the coercive consequences delimited for the different occasions will depend on the contexts where the therapist acts, and it is important that the reader knows those in force in his/her region. At the collective level, unethical behavior negatively interferes with the social recognition of the professional category, which ultimately affects its maintenance and harms the individuals who represent it.

A brief analysis of the recommendations contained in documents presented in codes of ethics directed to the psychologist indicates a prescriptive ethics, as defined by Dittrichi and Abib (2004), which describes how the professional *should behave*. However, many of the prescriptions present responses to be issued that will depend on the judgment of the psychologist and their previous analysis in each context. Each professional may interpret differently regulations or recommendations that, for example, describe principles such as "act in the law of least prejudice" or "share strictly necessary information about the client." In most cases, there will be a need for the professional's discretion as to what would be the least harm or what is strictly necessary to be shared about the client, in contexts of multiprofessional teams, judicial order issues, in the care of children and adolescents, etc.

Generic definitions as presented in the different ethical documents reflect, among other aspects, the complexity of the theme. Is it possible to describe point-to-point an ethical behavior to be issued by the professional before each specific situation? Could not information considered strictly necessary in a clinical case to be shared with a multiprofessional team be different in a similar case, but in another context or with another team?

Skinner proposed a model of ethics defined as relational (Vandenbergue, 2005) and plastic, impossible to be delimited by rigid standards (Dittrichi & Abib, 2004). This position indicates how necessary is the prior analysis of the psychologist who needs to make ethical decisions in the face of each situation in which their behavior should be issued.

For Skinner (1953/2000), deciding is a preliminary behavior to the act about which one decides. Analyzing (and predicting) the possible effects of a given response would increase the probability of achieving maximum reinforcement. Based on this, Dittrichi (2010) proposed a model of consequence analysis potentially useful for decision-making on some ethical issue. The following steps were considered: (1) categorize the consequences, (2) define the affected persons or groups, (3) define the selective effects of the consequences, and (4) define the temporal sequence of the consequences.

This analysis, conducted in each situation involving ethical issues, provides the psychologist with elements to assess the different controlling variables present in the situation and can contribute to their decision-making process. In this chapter, it is intended to present the ethical recommendations present in normative documents to the psychologist, delimited in the context of child psychotherapy, and raise questions for reflection that may contribute to part of the ethical decision-making process. The prescriptions were gathered and synthesized into five categories of responses, which highlight aspects considered important in the development of the work of the child analytic-behavioral therapist and will be presented below.

Theoretical and Technical Aptitude

According to the Ethical Principles of Psychologists and Code of Conduct (APA, 2017), it is the psychologist's responsibility to (a) know the guiding principles of the code of conduct and comply with it, (b) adopt methods and techniques that are recognized and grounded by science, and (c) provide service for demands for which he or she has received adequate training, experience, and advice, in order to ensure the quality of the work.

Before discussing the proposed recommendations, we reiterate the importance of psychologists being aware of what is prescribed by the codes of ethics, policies, and laws in force in their work environment and community, consulting them whenever necessary, and contacting the councils, associations, and professional support groups in their region for specific guidance when in doubt about how to conduct a situation. We emphasize that as a scientific community, we guide our work by agreement to the practices outlined in the peer review, and as a professional category acting in different societies, it should be noted that claiming ignorance of these recommendations and regulations is not enough to abolish responsibility, following the principle that to perform the activity is necessary to commit to a community that invested in their training so that their actions were possible.

With regard to the provision of quality services by child behavior analysts, it is important to highlight some aspects. It is necessary that the behavior analyst has a thorough knowledge of the principles and concepts of behavioral science as well as the intervention strategies and procedures recommended by it. If the therapist of this approach does not know, for example, how to correctly identify the possible functions of a behavior, he probably will not be able to perform an appropriate analysis of his client's behavioral pattern (Iwata & Dozier, 2008). Or, still, if he does not know how to predict the possible side effects of an extinction procedure (Skinner, 1953/2000), he may expose his client to an aversive condition, harmful to the treatment and, mainly, to his life.

When it comes to child psychotherapy, it also makes sense that the clinician should be skilled in proposing activities and strategies related to the child's universe, such as knowing how to play, knowing how to talk in language accessible to the child, knowing about potentially reinforcing games and activities, and especially that he or she likes children. What would it be like if a child started intervention with a child therapist and he, for lack of interest or ability, was not a reinforcer? A negative experience with a professional may not only hinder the intervention but also make it difficult for the child to be exposed again to another therapist and, even worse, to other professionals, such as doctors or teachers.

Finally, the importance of the psychotherapist knowing himself stands out. For Skinner (1974/1976a), self-knowledge is the ability of the individual to describe the controlling variables of his behavior. Knowing about oneself, being able to identify abilities or difficulties, contributes for the psychotherapist to be inclined to attend the demands with which he has more interest, facility, or experience, which would increase the probability of a quality intervention. As stated by Banaco, "the psychotherapist is also a person who has his history of reinforcement" (1993, p.75), and his thoughts and feelings should be taken into consideration.

Action for the Benefit of Children

According to APA guidelines (2017), the therapist should understand who his client is and what relationship to establish with each individual who may be involved with his client. The object of intervention of child psychotherapy is the child, and his protection and care are a priority – including legally provided – but the responsibility for him is his parents or legal representatives. The challenge will always be to act in benefit of the child, promoting practices that ensure their well-being and development, while the therapist should share information and guidelines necessary for parents, caregivers, and teachers, among others, to collaborate in this process.

In this context, it is essential to question in whose benefit is the demand brought to psychotherapy. Solomon (2013) investigated several examples of parents seeking intervention for children who do not meet their expectations, among them, homosexuals or transgender people. What should be done in these cases? How to act when the content of the complaint is the product of parental prejudice? Should the therapist, in this case, remain neutral or should he or she position himself or herself in some way?

Conducting interventions that aim to modify behavioral patterns by mere preference may not only diverge from the principles that guide the psychologist's practice but also contradict what is beneficial to the child. Prioritizing the child and its full development should be a basic premise to base any conduct of the child therapist.

Besides this issue, we observed in Holland (1978) the discussion about the specific relationship that a behavioral therapist can live with the people who undergo his interventions; many times the ones who define his objectives are not the clients but third parties. Analyzing these relationships becomes essential for the ethics of care.

It seems unreasonable, therefore, to establish a priori impediment relative to the attendance of people with whom the therapist already has some bond or to the establishment of a personal bond in the course of the intervention. However, it is fundamental that the therapist identifies (before and during) the effects of an intervention with these characteristics. There are situations in which the therapist has a personal bond established with the child's parents before the beginning of the intervention. What is the ethical conduct of the clinician in this context, initiate therapy or refer the child to another professional?

In practice, the therapist can choose how to act, provided that his conduct is the product of previous reflection on the different variables involved in each situation and their likely effects. It may be useful, for example, that by knowing the child's parents the therapist has access to variables of the context which he would not have if this relationship did not exist and whose lack of knowledge would hinder the progress of the intervention. On the other hand, it may be that a previous attachment of the child's parents to the therapist makes it difficult for the child to trust the therapist, for fear that what is open to him will be shared with his parents.

It may also be that the child is under coercive control in his home environment, which could imply at least two problems for the therapist. The first would be the therapist sharing aversive characteristics (Skinner, 1953/2000), due to establishing relationships with figures who adopt coercive practices, and the second would be the therapist having to intervene in the contingencies present in the home environment. Would a personal bond contribute to this intervention or hinder the therapist's management?

When it comes to the therapist-child bond, there are several variables that may interfere with the appropriate conduct of the intervention. In adult psychotherapy, although it is possible that the client establishes a strong bond with the therapist, in general, the adult is able to understand the specificity of this relationship. The therapist is also able to evaluate the possible interference of the bond with the client and may make this one of the objectives of his intervention (Kohlenberg & Tsai, 1991).

In child psychotherapy, however, it can be difficult for the child to understand the boundaries of the relationship. How can someone who is so nice and whom the child likes or trusts so much not be allowed, for example, to attend his home or birthday parties? The therapist may decide, on the other hand, to accept an invitation from the child for his birthday, but should not do so without first analyzing the situation. Variables that may be considered in making the decision are as follows: (a) Where did the invitation come from – are the parents and the child in agreement about the therapist's presence? (b) Does his presence fulfill part of the objectives of therapy (e.g., the child feels valued) or, oppositely, would it go against the intervention proposal, if he is facing a child with difficulties to hear "no"? In cases of this nature, the therapist may act in any direction, as long as he conducts a careful evaluation that foresees the probable effects of his conduct, as proposed by Dittrichi (2010). Again, the fundamental is that the therapist's decision is always based on what is beneficial to the child's therapy (and development).

Despite these considerations, although it is impossible for the therapist to be a *neutral* element, since he will establish a reinforcing history with the child, it will probably always be of greater contribution to the intervention to deal with variables that are accessible to his observation and evaluation. Experiencing new stories with the child in extra-therapeutic contexts may influence the therapist-child bond in such a way as to make it difficult to properly assess the variables that control the child's behavior and your own behavior.

Finally, Skinner (1953/2000) stated that psychotherapy aims to "reverse the behavioral changes that occur as a result of punishment" (p. 404) and that the therapist should configure himself as a nonpunitive audience. As stated by Vermes et al. (2007), the therapist should welcome the client without any criticism or judgment, and the selection for strategies involving positive reinforcement should be sovereign (Sidman, 1995; Skinner, 1953/2000). As Skinner (1953/2000) defined, in addition to the response reinforcement effect, the pleasure effect is also part of positive reinforcement contingencies. Thus, creating a context in which the child can have fun is an important step for both therapy and therapist to be reinforcing sources.

Exposing the child to potentially aversive situations, such as talking about difficult subjects, for example, requires careful planning by the therapist about the contingencies to be arranged. If the aversive effect is unavoidable, it is essential that the therapist plan additional strategies that potentiate alternative positive effects.

Share Information

Confidentiality and information sharing are issues of primary relevance in clinical practice. To address potential conflicts in situations of information protection or exposure, the APA (2017) states as guiding principles: "The primary obligation to take reasonable precautions to protect confidential information obtained, through or stored in any medium, recognizing that the extent and limits of confidentiality may be regulated by law or established by institutional, professional, or scientific relationship rules" (APA, 2017, art. 4.01). However, it is reserved the possibility of exposing the information in cases of patient consent, unless prohibited by law, and, when there is no consent, it is possible that this occurs in cases that the law requires or allows sharing in criteria of relevance. The Code of Conduct in 4.05, item b, lists four possibilities: (1) to promote necessary professional services; (2) to obtain appropriate professional consultation; (3) to protect the client/patient, psychologist, or others from harm; or (4) to obtain payment for services from a client/patient, in which case disclosure is limited to the minimum necessary to accomplish the purpose.

In child psychotherapy, issues regarding confidentiality tend to be frequent, first, because the therapist establishes a direct relationship with the child's parents, who expect frequent feedback from the therapist about aspects of the intervention. In general, parents seek therapy for their child because they identify something that concerns them and want it to improve. Parents have a right to information about their children. However, when starting the intervention in child therapy, the therapist makes a commitment to the child that whatever is talked about in that context will be a secret between them.

In addition, it is not uncommon that the therapist needs to relate to professionals from other areas who are part of the multiprofessional team. The exchange of information is common practice in these cases. But, what makes sense to share? How does one define what is strictly necessary information, following the recommendation of the Codes of Conduct?

Millenson (1967/1975) defined process as "what happens over time with significant aspects of behavior as a procedure is applied" (p. 56). Differentiating the content of what the child does in therapy, such as what he or she draws in front of an instruction, what he or she tells in a fantasy story, and comments he or she makes during play, from functions of these behaviors in relation to the chief complaints may help the therapist decide what to share with parents. It will probably always be more useful to share aspects of the process than to present data about the content of the activities performed. When a child verbalizes that "he doesn't like daddy because he is very angry or because he grounded him," the therapist can talk to the parents, for example, about the effect of coercive parenting practices, without necessarily describing the content of what the child did or said.

One must agree, however, that in situations in which psychotherapy is carried out with children with easily manageable complaints and cooperative parents, deciding on the confidentiality of information is usually a relatively simple task. On the other hand, there are situations in which the breach of confidentiality is mandatory, as a way to preserve the physical and emotional integrity of a child. In general, we observe that for decisions of this type, it is chosen to start from the principle of the least risk or harm and, especially, to ensure the protection of the child.

Examples of some situations like these are those involving suspected or confirmed sexual abuse and/or physical violence, neglect, maltreatment, and parental alienation. Although the decision is not always easy, either because the therapist is not sure of the facts or because it may involve precisely those people who are responsible for taking care of the child's life, the time variable for decision-making is primordial, since in these cases it determines the time of exposure of the child to the observed violence.

Acting quickly does not mean acting without caution. It is up to the psychotherapist to analyze the situation before choosing to break confidentiality and other measures. This analysis should include (a) a survey of the maximum possible variables that may contribute to the therapist's evaluation; (b) contact with members of the multiprofessional team (if any), in order to probe if there is similar suspicion; (c) contact (via telephone or website) with the body or association representing the professional class in the region, for guidance; and (d) supervision with an experienced therapist (if the therapist considers it necessary) or dialogue with colleagues who have experience with similar cases.

In spite of this, it is fundamental that the therapist knows that the investigative function of the cases does not fall to him/her. This function is generally performed by other social organs, public, or, if they exist in their realities and communities, by the Guardianship Councils and the Child and Youth Courts. The excess of caution, proper of the nature of the profession, can put the child at greater risk or even incur in punishment to the psychologist.

In situations in which the child therapist is requested to testify in court, it is important that he/she only provide information that is the result of objective procedures of data collection and analysis and that he/she only takes a position in favor of one side when he/she has sufficient information to justify his/her conduct. Otherwise, it is recommended that he or she be descriptive and neutral, so that the case can be investigated and judged by the responsible bodies.

Documents: Preparation and Care

Some associations and bodies responsible for the profession of psychologist may make it mandatory to record the intervention performed, in the form of a medical record. The medical record is a common document for health professionals and its purpose is to "facilitate patient care" (Farina, 1999, par.1). The information contained in it can be accessed by the patient, whenever requested, since the medical record belongs to the patient (Farina, 1999). In child psychotherapy, it does not make sense for parents to access all the information of the intervention, so the information that can be accessed at any time should be included in the record.

The recommendations of codes of ethics and conduct are usually concerned with talking about documentary records. In the publication of the APA (2017), we observed that functions are defined for the record that should guide the therapist's practice of recording. The documents produced from the notes and information collection in professional activity should have a scientific character and the purpose of: "(1) facilitate the provision of services by them or by other professionals later, (2) enable replication of planning and research analysis, (3) meet institutional requirements, (4) ensure billing and payment accuracy, and (5) ensure compliance with the law (APA, 2017, Art 6.01)." A good example of a medical record or the documentary record should contain a set of information whose purpose is to succinctly describe the work, covering the following items: (a) identification data, (b) assessment of the complaint and establishment of work objectives, (c) record of the evolution of the case and the procedures adopted, and (d) record of referral or closure (Conselho Federal de Psicologia, 2005). It should also contain the copy of additional documents that were written by the psychologist throughout the intervention.

The fundamental thing is that the therapist records the evolution of the case in a medical record or documentary record. The update of the record is decided by each therapist, depending on the criteria they use to define objectives and to evaluate the evolution of the case.

On this topic, it is worth mentioning the seminal study by Baer et al. (1968), which offered fundamental dimensions for applied research in behavior analysis and that could guide any intervention in this approach. Among the proposed guidelines are the selection and description of procedures based on science, the recording of the measures used, and the constant evaluation of the effects of the intervention on the individual's behavior. Child behavior-analytic therapists should consider these recommendations in the daily exercise of their work.

With regard to other documents that may be requested by the child's legal guardians or by judicial requests, it is necessary for the psychologist to follow the structures defined by the bodies that regulate the profession in their region. In general, the bodies define the types of documents and how the structure of the document should be in different cases. If, by chance, this does not occur in the reality of the therapist's profession, it is recommended that the therapist contact these bodies or associations, formally requesting guidance. Some examples of different documents are (a) statement, (b) attestation, (c) report, and (d) opinion (Conselho Federal de Psicologia, 2011). Each of these documents serves a specific purpose and should be written in clear and precise language, including only the information that is essential to fulfill the purpose of the requested document.

It is also reiterated that the documents produced by a psychologist must meet the scientific parameters of the area. To this end, it is strongly recommended that the therapist collect data in the most diverse situations and be parsimonious. Describing what was observed is different from inferring data from mere observation. Even if the therapist establishes working hypotheses, it only makes sense for him/her to describe them as a conclusion if he/she has obtained the data from experimentation, as described by Iwata and Dozier (2008). Otherwise, the therapist should record his observations and present possible hypotheses (when based on hard data) without subjective judgments.

The professional should also take care that the documents are stored in an appropriate place, preserving the confidentiality of the information. The information can be registered on paper or in computerized media, but it is essential that the access to it is protected. The documents must be available for inspection by the professional regulatory bodies, when requested. Finally, it is recommended, and for some regulatory bodies of the profession, mandatory, that the psychologist be responsible for the final destination of the confidential files, in order to ensure the privacy and identification data of his or her client (example: Conselho Federal de Psicologia, 2011).

Relating to Other Professionals

In most cases the child therapist will relate to other professionals, psychologists, or from other professions throughout the interventions. Therefore, the assumptions of multiprofessional teamwork are relevant repertoires of support and guidance to therapists' conduct. It should be emphasized that teams should ensure constant communication and organize their activities based on scientific methodology. In addition, it is part of the work to contact a previous professional, if there is one and if it is possible, either by request of those responsible for the child or by decision of the psychologist himself; in the latter, those responsible for the child must agree. The collection of information about the case, including what was the complaint that led the child to the previous clinician, what was the methodology of his work, what effects he observed during treatment, and what was his general view about the case, can contribute to the current therapist's analysis and planning for the intervention.

In the context of child care by multiprofessional team, communication with professionals should be constant, respecting the limits of confidentiality of the intervention. As already presented, one should share only the information that is relevant to the general understanding of the case, without providing details that unnecessarily expose the child or communicating aspects of the therapist-client relationship that will not lead to any benefit for the progress of the intervention.

Finally, the recognition of the specificity of their work and the scope of their intervention is necessary so that psychotherapists do not assume responsibilities for which they are not qualified, and, if they observe that they are facing a demand for which their specific knowledge is not adequate, they should take responsibility for referring it to the appropriate professionals. In cases of children with difficulties in different areas, it is important that the therapist evaluate which professional can best meet the demand and make the referral.

Conclusion

This chapter aimed to present some ethical issues pertinent to the context of child psychotherapy. The main recommendations from normative documents were synthesized in the following categories: (a) being theoretically and technically able; (b) acting for the benefit of the child; (c) sharing information; (d) drafting, keeping, and forwarding documents; and (e) relating with other professionals. An attempt was made to define these actions of the therapist, considering the way they relate to the daily life of the child psychotherapist.

The aspects raised demonstrate the importance of the psychologist being aware of which behaviors are defined as ethical within their category and professional regulatory body and demonstrate, above all, the need for an analysis of the multiple variables involved in each ethical decision-making situation. As Vandenbergue (2005) highlighted, analyzing contexts "imposes a relational ethic on the therapist, in which the clinician has responsibility not only for the client, but also for the contexts in which their actions and the effects of their actions have relevance" (p. 64).

In the face of ethical conflicts, the professional will benefit from guidance from councils, associations, and other bodies that come to regulate the profession in their context and region, from contact with other colleagues who have experience with similar situations, and with members of the multiprofessional team (if any). Monitoring news on related themes contributes to the improvement of the clinician's repertoire. Newspapers, bulletins, and communications from professional support and regulatory bodies, as well as the websites of these institutions, generally contain constant and updated information on ethical issues in the daily life of the professional. A varied repertoire on the part of the therapist develops in the exposure to different contingencies and contributes to their conduct being.

The survey of issues that may contribute to therapist decision-making suggests that Skinner's proposals for psychotherapy (1953/2000) and for situations involving the teaching of skills (1968/1972) may assist child therapists in acting ethically in the different circumstances of their daily professional life. Examples of these proposals are (a) the indication of the use of massive positive reinforcement in detriment to aversive control as the basis of intervention strategies, (b) the suggestion for the therapist to evaluate the effects of the client's behavior in the context in which he/she is inserted, (c) the recommendation for the therapist to establish himself/herself as a nonpunitive audience, (d) the notion of multidetermination of behavior and the need for the identification of the several variables that control behavior, (e) the indication of performance recording, and (f) the constant measurement of the intervention effects, to name a few.

Knowing the guiding principles of behavioral science and basing application strategies on them will increase the likelihood that the child therapist will adopt ethical conduct. And finally, as stated by Dittrichi and Abib (2004) "if behavior analysis is supported by a philosophy – radical behaviorism – which includes an ethical system, it is expected that analysts seek in this system the guidelines for their interventions" (p. 432).

References

American Psychological Association (2017). *Ethical Principles of Psychologists and Code of Conduct*. Washington, DC: American Psychological Association.

Baer, D., Wolf, M., & Risley, T. R. (1968). Some current dimensions of applied behavior analysis. *Journal of Applied Behavior Analysis, 1*, 91–97.

Banaco, R. (1993). O impacto do atendimento sobre a pessoa do terapeuta. *Temas em Psicologia, 2*, 71–79.

Conselho Federal de Psicologia. (2005). Resolução CFP n° 010/2005. Código de Ética Profissional do Psicólogo.

Dittrichi, A. (2010). Análise de consequências como procedimento para decisões éticas. *Revista Perspectivas em Análise do Comportamento, 1*, 44–54. http://pepsic.bvsalud.org/scielo.php?script=sci_abstract&pid=S2177-35482010000100007&lng=pt&nrm=iso

Dittrichi, A., & Abib, J. A. D. A. (2004). O Sistema Ético Skinneriano e Conseqüências para a Prática dos Analistas do Comportamento. *Psicologia: Reflexão e Crítica, 17*, 427–433.

Farina, A. (1999). *Prontuário Médico*. http://portal.cfm.org.br/index.php?option=com_content&id=20462:prontuario-medico

Ferreira, M. C. B. (2018). *Valores secundários em Skinner e justiça social: Compromissos éticos para a educação (Dissertação de mestrado)*. Universidade Estadual de Londrina.

Gianfaldoni, M. H. T. A. (2005). *A educação como prática cultural ética: Uma leitura possível das propostas de B. F. Skinner (Tese de doutorado)*. Pontifícia Universidade Católica de São Paulo.

Holland, J.G. (1978). Behaviorism: Part of the problem or part of the solution? *Journal of Applied Behavior Analysis, 11*, 163–174. https://doi.org/10.1901/jaba.1978.11-163

Iwata, B. A., & Dozier, C. L. (2008). Clinical application of functional analysis methodology. *Behavior Analysis in Practice, 1*, 3–9.

Kohlenberg, R. J., & Tsai, M. (1991). Functional analytic psychotherapy: Creating intense and curative therapeutic relationships. *Plenum Press*. https://doi.org/10.1007/978-0-387-70855-3

La Taille, Y. (2006). *Moral e ética*. Dimensões intelectuais e afetivas. Porto Alegre: Artmed.

Millenson, J. R. (1975). *Princípios de análise do comportamento*. (A. A. Souza & D. Rezende Trads.). Coordenada (Original paper published in 1967).

Sidman, M. (1995). *Coerção e suas implicações*. (M. A. Andery & T. M. Sério, Trads.). Psy II.

Skinner, B. F. (1972). *Tecnologia do ensino*. (R. Azzi Trad.). E.P.U, EDUSP. (Original paper published in 1968).

Skinner, B. F. (1976a) *About behaviorism*. Vintage Books Edition. (Original paper published in 1974).

Skinner, B.F. (1976b). *Beyond freedom and dignity*. Penguin books Ltda (Original paper published in 1971).

Skinner, B. F. (2000). *Ciência e comportamento humano* (J. C. Todorov & R. Azzi, Trads.). Martins Fontes. (Original paper published in 1953).

Solomon, A. (2013). Longe da árvore. In *Pais, filhos e a busca da identidade*. Companhia das Letras.

Vandenbergue, L. (2005). Uma ética behaviorista radical para a terapia comportamental. *Revista Brasileira de Terapia Comportamental e Cognitiva, 1*, 55–66.

Vermes, J., Zamignani, D., & Kovac, R. (2007). A relação terapêutica no atendimento clinico em ambiente extraconsultório. In D. R. Zamignani, R. Kovac, & J. S. Vermes (Eds.), *A clínica de portas abertas*. Paradigma. ESETec.

Index

A
Acceptance and commitment therapy (ACT), 3, 93–95, 98–101, 171
Assessment tools, 128

B
Behavioral cusps, 20–22, 29
Behavior analysis, 1, 2, 11, 12, 17–29, 33, 74, 75, 84, 105, 106, 114, 125, 145, 153, 157, 158, 163, 169, 177, 194, 197
Behavior therapist, 107, 109
Behavior therapy, 105, 114, 123
Biological bases, 23, 39

C
Case formulation, 11, 46, 52, 135, 142, 167, 170, 180, 181
Child behavior-analytic therapy, 1–7, 141
Child behavior therapy, 84, 108
Child development, 17, 27, 29, 33, 36, 46, 83–86, 134
Childhood psychiatric disorders, 136, 139
Child psychotherapy, 1, 3, 5, 81, 106, 117, 159, 189–192, 194, 196
Children therapy, 3, 5–7, 10–12, 14, 46, 47, 52, 81, 84, 85, 87, 93–101
Clinical assessment, 45–53
Clinical behavior analysis, 1–7, 45–53, 84, 86, 91, 139–141, 145–148, 155, 158, 175–185, 187–197
Clinical behavior analysis for children, 1–7, 45–53, 84, 86, 91, 139–141, 145–148, 155, 158, 175–185, 187–197
Clinical case formulation, 170, 180

Clinically relevant behavior (CRB), 50, 81, 108–113, 170
Contextual therapy, 93
Critical period, 25
Culture, 9, 19, 26, 70, 83, 140, 146, 159, 168, 187

D
Developmental milestones, 18–20, 29

E
Early childhood, 25–28, 99, 177
Ethics, 3, 16, 128, 187–190, 194, 196
Evidence-based treatment, 66, 67

F
Family intervention, 73
Family-school relationship, 126
Family therapy, 77, 163–165, 167, 169
Family treatment, 51, 52, 75, 77, 127
Functional analytic psychotherapy (FAP), 3, 105–115, 118, 170
Functional play, 82, 84–86, 91

G
Goodness-of-fit, 41

I
Interdisciplinarity, 134, 135
Interdisciplinary intervention, 133–142
Intervention with children, 114, 181

L
Levels of therapeutic intervention, 117–124
Life skills, 181–183

M
Maturation, 7, 17, 22–25, 35, 133
Mental disorders, 37, 99, 147
Mental health, 2, 13, 16, 27, 40, 70, 72, 76, 77, 134, 135, 142
Multidisciplinary, 15, 73, 129, 130, 141
Multidisciplinary intervention, 141

N
Neurodevelopment, 133–134, 140

P
Parental guidance, 4, 52, 136, 140, 145–159, 163, 171, 180, 181
Parental training, 4, 137, 145–159
Parent-children interaction, 41, 149–158
Parenting, 5, 36, 41, 42, 49, 51, 52, 74, 77, 145, 147, 148, 150, 151, 155–158, 182, 193
Parent training, 48, 74, 77, 145, 153, 155–157
Playful assessment, 3, 4, 14, 46, 50, 75, 85, 101, 179
Play therapy, 81
Prevention, 13, 28, 29, 70, 75–77, 176
Problem-solving style, 119–120

R
Radical behaviorism, 1, 2, 82, 93, 105, 142, 197
Relapse prevention, 73, 76, 181–183, 185

T
Team working, 135
Temperament, 33, 36, 38–42
Therapeutic assessment, 47
Therapeutic discharge, 175–177, 180, 184
Therapeutic goals, 45–53, 105, 128, 130, 168, 176, 181
Therapeutic interaction, 114, 118
Therapeutic myths, 47
Therapeutic process, 3–5, 7, 10–16, 46–50, 52, 86, 88, 110, 113, 124–126, 169–171, 176–184
Therapeutic tools, 3, 4, 180
Therapist-school relationship, 129
Therapist's role, 10, 15
Therapy with children, 7, 106–107

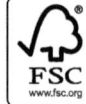

MIX
Papier aus verantwortungsvollen Quellen
Paper from responsible sources
FSC® C105338

If you have any concerns about our products,
you can contact us on
ProductSafety@springernature.com

In case Publisher is established outside the EU,
the EU authorized representative is:
**Springer Nature Customer Service Center GmbH
Europaplatz 3, 69115 Heidelberg, Germany**

Printed by Libri Plureos GmbH
in Hamburg, Germany